KNEE
REPLACEMENT

KNEE REPLACEMENT

THIRD EDITION

SKS Marya

MS(Orthopedics, PGI) DNB(Orthopedics)
MCh(Orthopedics, Liverpool) FRCS(England) DSc(Amity University)

Chairman and Chief Surgeon (Pan Max) and Chief Advisor
Max Institute of Musculoskeletal Sciences and Orthopaedics
New Delhi and Gurugram, India

Rajiv Thukral

MS DNB FCPS(Orthopedics)

Director Orthopedics and Head, Joint Replacement Program
Yatharth Group of Hospitals, Faridabad, Delhi NCR
Faridabad, Haryana, India

Foreword

Sam Oussedik

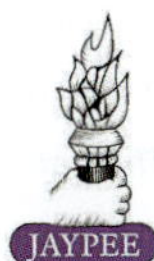

JAYPEE BROTHERS MEDICAL PUBLISHERS

The Health Sciences Publisher

New Delhi | London

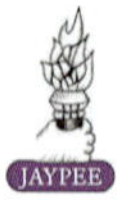
JAYPEE **Jaypee Brothers Medical Publishers (P) Ltd**

Headquarters
EMCA House
23/23-B, Ansari Road, Daryaganj
New Delhi 110 002, India
Landline: +91-11-23272143, +91-11-23272703
+91-11-23282021, +91-11-23245672
E-mail: jaypee@jaypeebrothers.com

Corporate Office
Jaypee Brothers Medical Publishers (P) Ltd.
4838/24, Ansari Road, Daryaganj
New Delhi 110 002, India
Phone: +91-11-43574357
Fax: +91-11-43574314
E-mail: jaypee@jaypeebrothers.com

Overseas Office
JP Medical Ltd.
83, Victoria Street, London
SW1H 0HW (UK)
Phone: +44-20 3170 8910
Fax: +44(0)20 3008 6180
E-mail: info@jpmedpub.com

Website: www.jaypeebrothers.com
Website: www.jaypeedigital.com

Inquiries for bulk sales may be solicited at: jaypee@jaypeebrothers.com

***Knee Replacement* / SKS Marya, Rajiv Thukral**

First Edition: 2007

Third Edition: **2025**

ISBN: 978-93-6616-390-1

Printed at: Samrat Offset Pvt. Ltd.

DEDICATED TO

Shivan and Shaman my friends who also happen to be our sons.
My wife Mohini for her support for all three of us.

— **SKS Marya**

Aman and Aaditya, for their unhesitating sacrifice of our father-son time together; and Kavita, for her unwavering faith in me and my abilities.

— **Rajiv Thukral**

Foreword

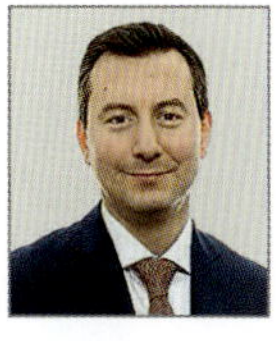

Sam Oussedik BSc FRCS (Tr and Orth)
Consultant Orthopedic Surgeon and Head
University College London Hospital NHS Trust
Honorary Associate Professor, University College London
London, United Kingdom

Total knee arthroplasty is one of the most effective surgical procedures for relieving pain and improving function, leading to better quality and, indeed, greater quantity of life. With such excellent results achievable, the pressure is on the surgical team to deliver, time after time after time.

How to achieve the best results for our patients? Careful preoperative assessment to identify risk factors for complications, preoperative planning to mitigate their effects and create a detailed surgical plan, in-depth anatomical knowledge to provide the correct surgical approach to deformity correction and soft-tissue balancing—no more and no less than required, immaculate surgical technique to deliver the surgical plan, empathy and motivation in equal parts to lead our patients through their difficult yet vital postoperative rehabilitation.

The knowledge required to address each of these points is contained within this excellent tome. Together with the hands-on training that forms the cornerstone of our professional development, it will allow the surgeon to provide safe, effective care when carrying out total knee arthroplasty procedures.

To be a surgeon is to commit to lifelong learning and self-improvement: "Study," "Practice," "Reflect," "Repeat". This is our mantra. This book will be a companion on your journey toward surgical proficiency. I am sure you will find time spent with it most rewarding.

Preface to the Third Edition

After the overwhelming response to the first and second editions of this volume, our colleagues (juniors and peers) suggested an updated version to include the effect of modern trends and technology on the practice of arthroplasty. We were also aware that the current generation arthroplasty surgeon must not only be well versed with the basics of knee replacement (a hallmark of our first edition), but also the way technology is shaping modern understanding, preoperative workup, anesthetic techniques, surgical approaches, and rehabilitation strategies.

The new 3rd edition *"Knee Replacement"* was thus conceptualized and comes with chapters on alignment philosophies, deep vein thrombosis (DVT) prophylaxis, implant options (including unicompartmental, bicompartmental, and bicruciate sparing knees), and technology (navigation, robotics, 3D printing, patient specific instrumentation, and custom implants) to achieve the goal of personalized knee replacement.

The new chapters on compartmental total knee arthroplasty (TKA) and technology in TKA give insights into the present-day trends and options available to restore alignment, balance, native anatomy, and function. Among all these shifts in alignment-based, technology-assisted implantation philosophy, we must remind one and all that this surgery continues to be an artful soft tissue and bone balancing act.

1st January, 2025
New Delhi

SKS Marya
Rajiv Thukral

Preface to the First Edition

Knee replacement is here to stay and like every new and exciting technology it catches the fancy of every aspiring young orthopod. Any why not?

However, it needs to be appreciated that to understand the techniques and offer relief to millions of affected people the surgery must be performed correctly and systematically again and again and again. This requires extensive learning both on the study table and the operation table not to mention prolonged interactions with patients in the wards and outpatient department.

Over a period of time, a large number of young colleagues appeared quite uncertain as to which book to consult and to get a fair idea of knee replacement surgery. Either the volumes were extensive or difficult to understand or for a beginner the details in surgical technique manual were inadequate.

The book was hence conceived as a step-by-step teaching guide for the aspiring and young joint replacement surgeons. Colored pictures of the techniques have been liberally used to try and make things look easy and sequential. In addition, preoperative, intraoperative, and postoperative aspects have been broadly covered.

In nutshell, the message is to choose one system and one methodical approach. Soft tissues must be respected, and it is important to remember that knee replacement is more of a soft-tissue procedure and not a case of cutting the bones.

29th August, 2006 **SKS Marya**
New Delhi

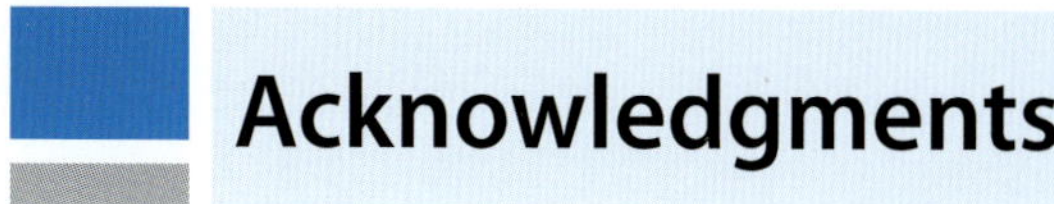

Acknowledgments

A few pictures have been taken from the Johnson and Johnson website and we are grateful for the same.

Contents

Chapter 1	History and Basics	1
Chapter 2	Relevant Surgical Anatomy	5
Chapter 3	Biomechanics and Alignment	11
Chapter 4	Getting Started: Implant Systems and Designs	17
Chapter 5	Surgical Approaches	19
Chapter 6	Indications and Contraindications	27
Chapter 7	Preoperative Preparation	31
Chapter 8	Preoperative Clinical Assessment	35
Chapter 9	Radiology and Templating	41
Chapter 10	Scoring	44
Chapter 11	Surgical Technique: Standard Knee	49
Chapter 12	Surgical Technique: Varus Deformity	74
Chapter 13	Surgical Technique: Valgus Deformity	78
Chapter 14	Surgical Technique: Flexion Deformity	85
Chapter 15	Surgical Technique: Bone Defect Management	90
Chapter 16	Surgical Technique: Recurvatum Deformity	95
Chapter 17	Surgical Technique: Fused Knee Takedown	100
Chapter 18	Postoperative Period	105
Chapter 19	Accelerated Physiotherapy Protocol	110
Chapter 20	Follow-up	112
Chapter 21	Thromboprophylaxis Update	114
Chapter 22	Complications	121

Chapter 23	Issues	127
Chapter 24	Current Day Economics of Total Knee Arthroplasty	133
Chapter 25	Compartmental Knee Arthroplasty	138
Chapter 26	Technology Today	154
Index		171

Chapter 1

History and Basics

Knee arthroplasty owes its origin to resection and resection-interposition techniques. Fergusson performed the first resection knee arthroplasty for arthritis in 1861, and Verneuil performed the first interposition arthroplasty in 1863 (using a flap of joint capsule between the resected bone ends). Other interposition materials used over time included skin, fat, muscle, and chromatized pig bladder. These grafts had limited success in ankylosed knees, but not in arthritis.

The first mold hemiarthroplasty (replacement of surfaces with a metallic mold) of the knee was attempted by Campbell and Boyd in 1940, and Smith-Petersen in 1942, but with limited success in pain relief. Tibial hemiarthroplasty was also attempted by McKeever and MacIntosh unsuccessfully. All these failed early due to loosening and severe pain.

The first true femoral and tibial articular replacement (incidentally *metal-on-metal*) happened in the 1950s as hinged implants developed by Walldius and Shiers. The GUEPAR hinge was later developed, followed by the Spherocentric knee and the Kinematic rotating hinge in 1981 **(Fig. 1)**. These designs also failed, possibly due to improper understanding of knee kinematics, infection, and loosening.

In 1971, Gunston reported his results with the polycentric knee (based on the concepts of Charnley's low-friction hip arthroplasty), introducing the concept of "femoral rollback" **(Fig. 2)**. These knees had improved kinematics; but failed due to inadequate fixation. This was followed by the Geomedic knee (1973), the Imperial College/London Hospital (ICLH) design (Freeman and Swanson), and the Duocondylar knee.

The total condylar prosthesis (by Insall and others) was subsequently developed at the Hospital for Special Surgery in 1973,

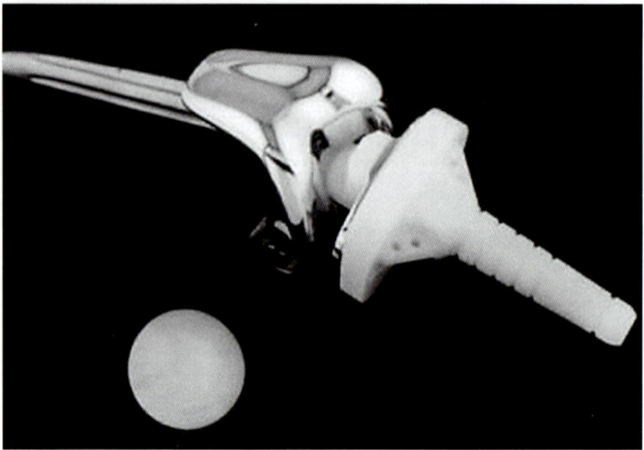

FIG. 1: The kinematic rotating hinge knee prosthesis.

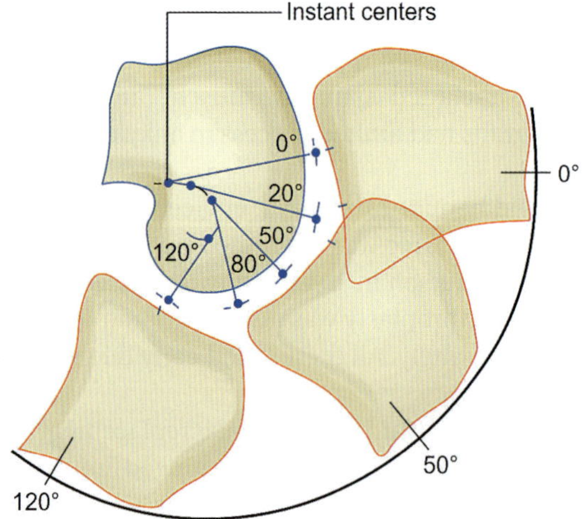

FIG. 2: Changing instant center of rotation of the knee.

for which Ranawat et al. reported survivorships of 94% at 15 years follow-up **(Fig. 3)**. This has set the standard for survivorship of all present-day total knee arthroplasty (TKA) prostheses. Concurrently, the Duopatellar knee (the first tricompartment knee, with anterior flanging for patellar articulation and cruciate-retention) was developed, which evolved into the Kinematic prosthesis, widely used in the 1980s. However, all these designs had problems of limited flexion, which was corrected by Insall–Burnstein designs in 1978 (by incorporating a central cam mechanism to induce femoral rollback), thereby improving range of flexion.

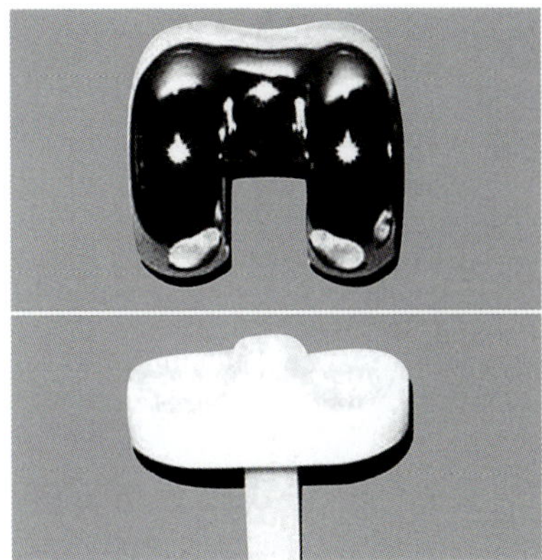
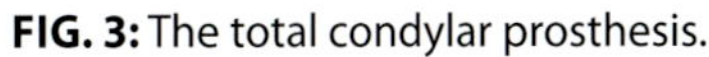

FIG. 3: The total condylar prosthesis.

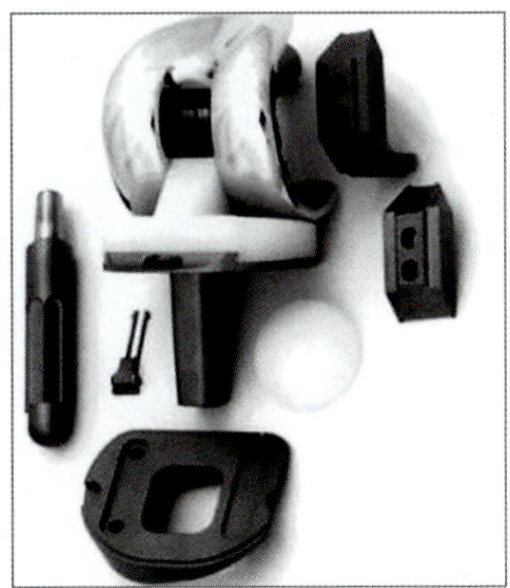

FIG. 4: Constrained condylar knee prosthesis.

The constrained condylar knee (CCK) was thereafter developed by Insall **(Fig. 4)**. The enlarged central tibial insert post constrained it against the medial and lateral walls of a deepened central femoral component box, thus paving the way for use of this design for difficult primary [extreme valgus deformity and medial collateral ligament (MCL) insufficiency] and revision arthroplasty (bone loss and instability).

The first mobile-bearing knee originated from the Oxford knee designed by Goodfellow and O'Conner in 1976 as a bicondylar knee, with totally congruent tibial polyethylene inserts (menisci) that were free to move on a polished metal tibial base plate. Thereafter, Beuchel and others developed the low contact stress (LCS) design, which was increasingly used, especially in younger patients **(Fig. 5)**.

Resurfacing of only one knee compartment was introduced by McKeever in the 1950s (metal tibial hemiarthroplasty), but suffered early failures, due to pain and loosening. Marmor developed his version in the 1970s (an anatomically-shaped flat, all-polyethylene component) with reasonable success **(Fig. 6)**. Subsequently, metal-backed components were developed and successfully implanted.

The present-day concept is to use prosthesis according to the type and severity of arthritis, and the associated deformity and laxity. The golden rule for the beginner is to acquaint oneself with one specific implant system, and to undertake TKA in knees with relatively mild deformity; and then gradually extend his/her skillset to tackle knees with complexity and severe deformity.

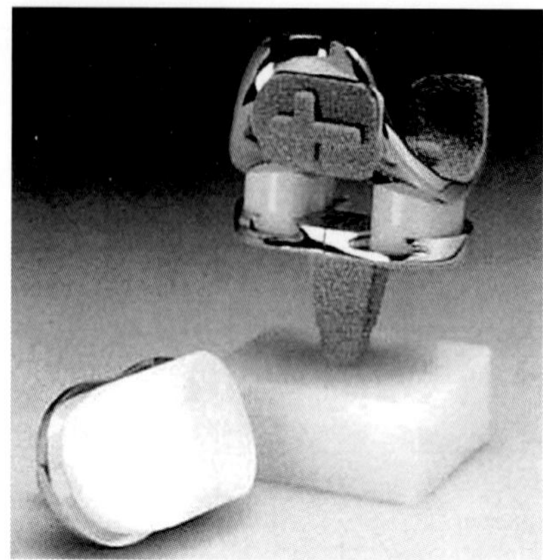

FIG. 5: The low contact stress (LCS) design.

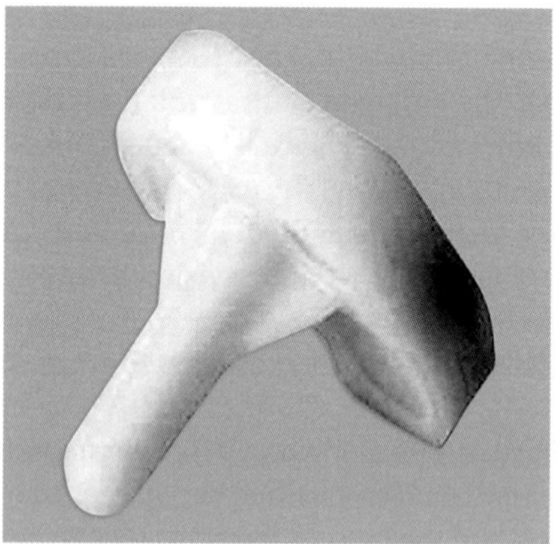

FIG. 6: All-poly tibial component.

Many new prosthetic materials (ceramics), designs (mobile-bearing, hi-flex), bearing surfaces (metal-metal or ceramic-poly), and binding options (hydroxyapatite-coating) have been researched, however, the tried and tested should be the method of choice for the early learners.

Chapter 2

Relevant Surgical Anatomy

Good knowledge of relevant anatomy is the prerequisite for a good surgical approach, dissection, surgical technique, and eventual outcome. This includes a thorough detailed study of bones, ligaments, muscles, and neurovascular structures around the knee joint.

OSTEOLOGY

The bony landmarks include the following:

- *Femur:* Intercondylar notch, relation of femoral canal to the notch, interepicondylar line, anterior intercondylar line, posterior intercondylar line, and distal femoral anatomical axis.
- *Tibia:* Tibial tubercle, tibial anatomical axis, posteromedial and posterolateral tibial surfaces, and insertion of posterior cruciate ligament (PCL) on tibia.
- *Patella:* Patella position, thickness, inclination, and patellar facets.

SOFT TISSUES

Knowledge of the soft tissues (viz., ligaments, both intra- and extra-articular, and muscles) is paramount to balancing the operated knee **(Fig. 1)**. The salient points are given in the following text.

Ligaments

- *Anterior cruciate ligament (ACL):* Origin, insertion, thickness, and functional integrity.
- *Posterior cruciate ligament:* Origin, insertion, thickness, and functional integrity.

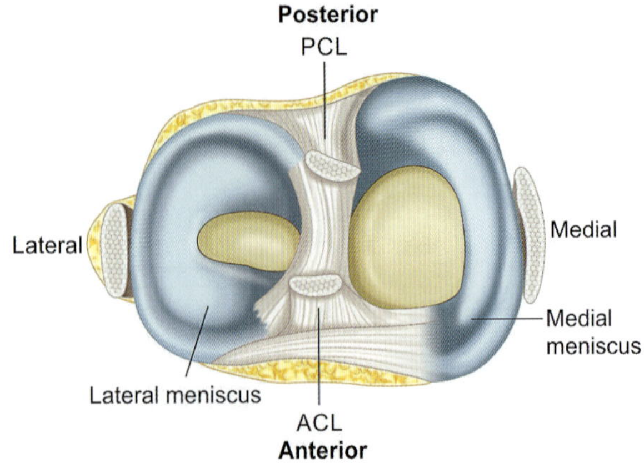

FIG. 1: Cross-sectional anatomy demonstrating position of knee menisci and ligaments.

(ACL: anterior cruciate ligament; PCL: posterior cruciate ligament)

- *Medial collateral ligament (MCL):* Origin, insertion, superficial portion, deep portion, attrition in valgus and tension in varus, and relation to medial meniscus.
- *Lateral collateral ligament (LCL):* Origin, insertion, attrition in varus and tension in valgus, relation to lateral meniscus and popliteus tendon.
- *Posterior capsule:* Relation to popliteus, hamstring tendons, popliteal vessels, and nerves.

Muscle Forces (Figs. 2 and 3)

- *Extensor mechanism:* Vastus lateralis, intermedius, medialis and obliquus, and tendon-muscle intersection.
- *Hamstrings:* Biceps femoris, semitendinosus and semimembranosus, and relation of the biceps tendon to the lateral popliteal nerve (LPN).
- *Popliteus tendon:* Origin, insertion, relation to lateral meniscus, and LCL.

Neurovascular Anatomy (Fig. 4)

Blood Supply

The knee is very vascular, and is supplied by a vascular plexus contributed by the following:

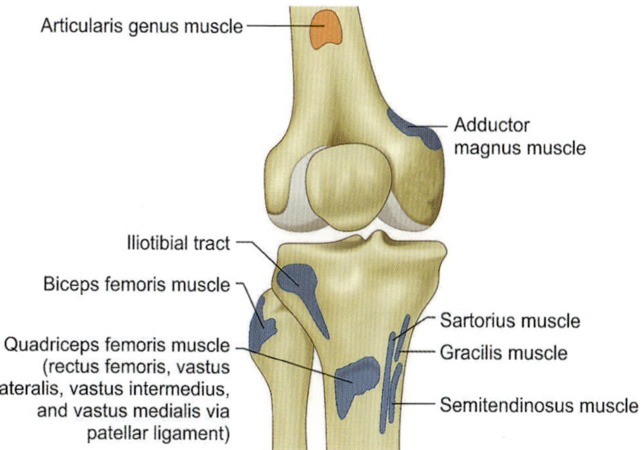

FIG. 2: Relevant surgical anatomy of the knee.

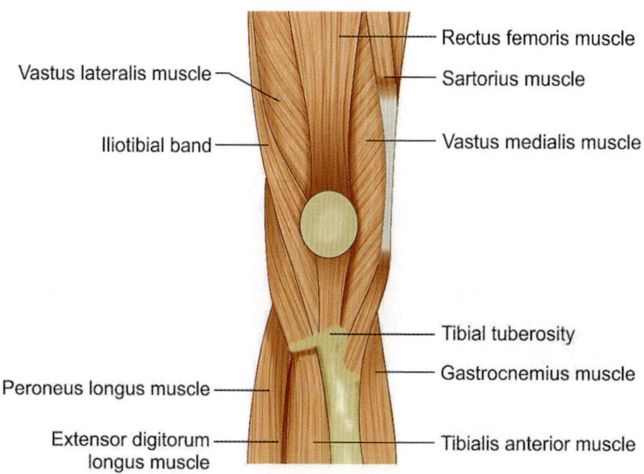

FIG. 3: Anterior muscular anatomy of the knee.

- Medial superior genicular;
- Lateral superior genicular;
- Middle genicular;
- Medial inferior genicular (passing deep to MCL, 2 cm distal to joint line);
- Lateral inferior genicular (passing deep to LCL at level of joint line);
- Descending branch of lateral circumflex femoral (LCF);
- Descending genicular branch of femoral artery (FA); and

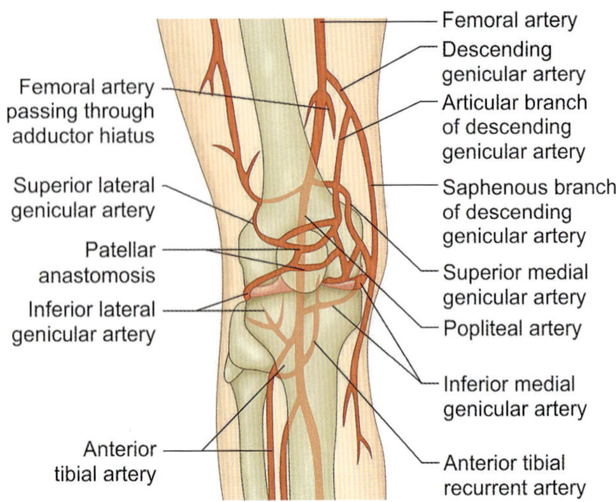

FIG. 4: Vascular anatomy around the knee.

- Recurrent vessels from the anterior tibial, posterior tibial (posterior tibial recurrent), circumflex fibular, and anterior tibial recurrent vessels.

The major offenders during intraoperative bleeding are the middle genicular (superficially) and the medial and lateral inferior genicular vessels (deep). *Knowledge of their relative anatomy ensures coagulation at the time of dissection, reducing intra- and postoperative blood loss, and postoperative hematoma formation.* Further, extreme care must be exercised during posterior capsule and PCL dissection, as the popliteal vessels lie immediately posterior.

Nerve Supply (Figs. 5 and 6)

Minor nerves are cut during dissection (the infrapatellar branch of the saphenous nerve), but the nerve courses that need to be studied include those of the following:

- *Tibial nerve:* Originating as the posterior branch of the sciatic (at the apex of the popliteal fossa), it passes superficial to the popliteus muscle (passing the popliteal artery from lateral to medial) and the soleus, deep to the gastrocnemius, sending branches to its medial and lateral heads, and the posterior cutaneous nerve of the calf, which travels along the course of the short saphenous vein.

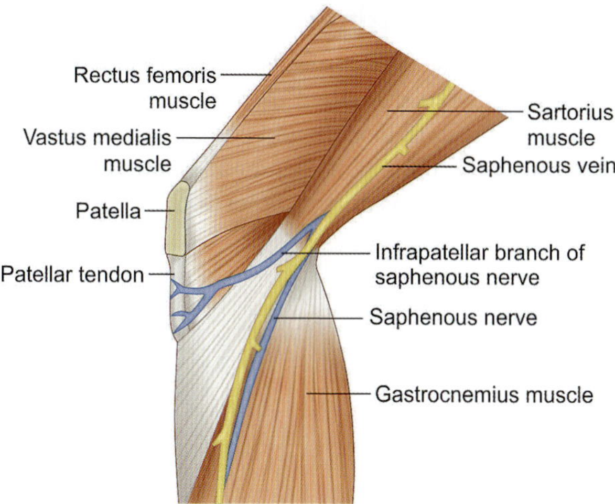

FIG. 5: Anteromedial nervous anatomy of the knee.

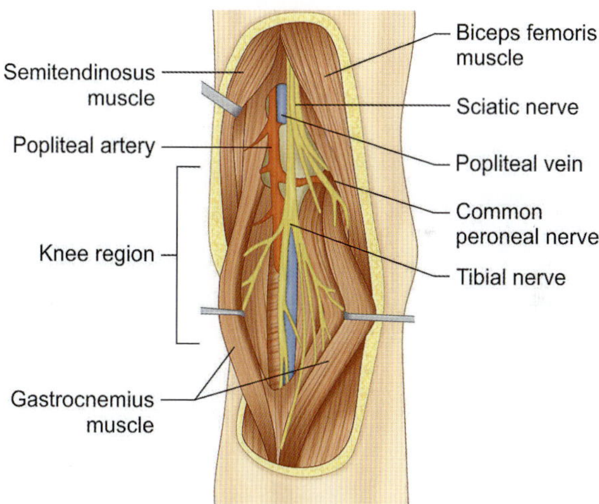

FIG. 6: Posterior nervous anatomy of the knee.

- *Lateral popliteal nerve (common peroneal nerve):* Originating along with the tibial nerve at the apex of the popliteal fossa, and traveling under the belly of the biceps femoris, curving around the neck of the fibula anteriorly, supplying the peroneal muscles. This nerve has the danger of being stretched during *valgus correction* as it is relatively fixed between the sciatic notch and the fibular neck.

Altered Anatomy in Arthritis

The anatomy of these structures is altered in deformities, and this variation has been described in brief during the appropriate sections on varus, valgus, flexion, and combined deformities. These may slightly alter the bone cuts, ligament balancing methods, and neurovascular implications during dissection.

Chapter 3

Biomechanics and Alignment

NORMAL KNEE

Kinematics

Knee motion during gait has been extensively studied and has been found to involve predominantly flexion and extension, some rotation, and minimal abduction and adduction. Stresses arising due to failure to account for these complex motions have led to the failure of many knee designs, and continuing emergence of newer anatomical designs.

Types of Alignment

"Normal" Coronal Alignment

- *Mechanical axis of the lower limb*: It is defined as a line drawn on a standing long leg anteroposterior (AP) roentgenogram, from the center of the femoral head to the center of the talar dome **(Fig. 1)**.
- This is different from the individual bone axes. Normally, this mechanical axis passes through or near the center of the knee joint. This axis is in 3° of valgus from the vertical axis of the body while standing in two-legged stance. When the mechanical axis lies lateral to the knee joint center on standing, the knee is in mechanical valgus, and vice versa.
- *Femur—anatomical axis*: It passes along the femoral shaft axis (pyriform fossa to intercondylar notch).
- *Tibia—anatomical axis*: It passes along the tibial shaft axis (intercondylar notch to tibial plafond center).
- *Femur—mechanical axis*: It passes from center of femoral head to center of intercondylar notch.

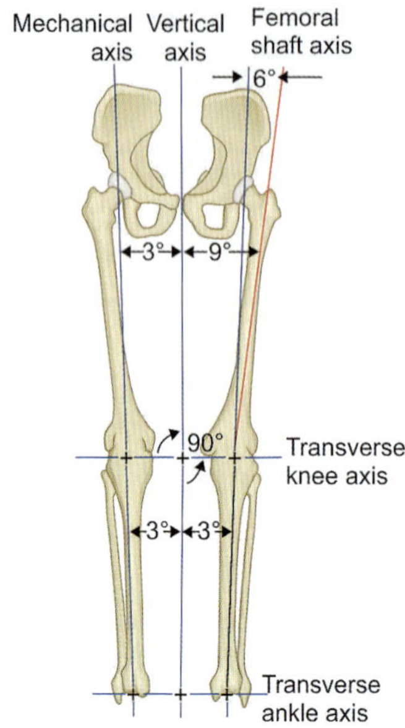

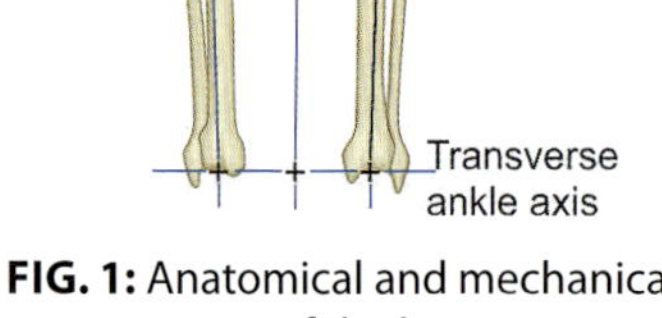

FIG. 1: Anatomical and mechanical axes of the knee.

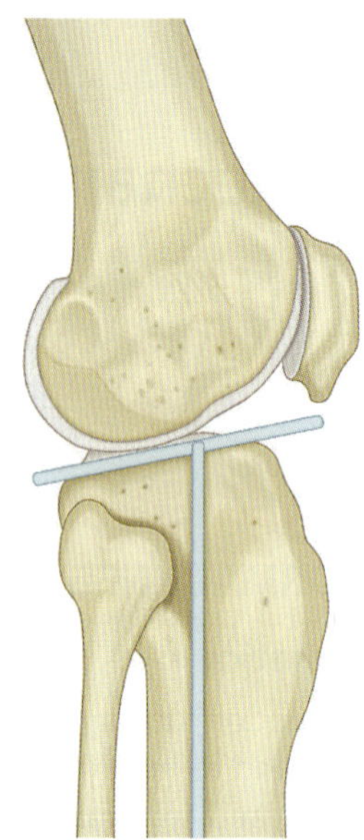

FIG. 2: Posterior tibial slope.

- *Tibia—mechanical axis*: It passes from center of tibial plateau to the center of tibial plafond. This usually corresponds to the tibial anatomical axis (unless there is tibial deformity).

"Normal" Sagittal Alignment

There is a "normal" posterior tibial slope of 7–10° (menisci correct this to 3°) **(Fig. 2)**.

Normally, the anatomical axes of the femur and the tibia form a valgus angle of 6° (±2°). In a "normal" knee, the tibial articular surface is in 3° varus to the mechanical axis, and the distal femoral surface is in a corresponding 9° valgus to the mechanical axis. 6° of variance therefore exists between the anatomical and mechanical femoral axes. Thus also, there is a medial proximal tibial angle (mPTA), lateral distal femoral angle (LDFA), and hip-knee-ankle angle (HKA).

Eckhoff, Bach et al. introduced the **coronal plane alignment of the knee (CPAK) classification** to define the "individual" knee alignment based on the relationship between the arithmetic (corrected) HKA (mPTA – LDFA) and the joint line obliquity angle (JLA) (mPTA + LDFA). The arithmetic HKA may lead to a varus, neutral, or valgus angle. Similarly, the JLA may have an apex distal, neutral, or apex proximal angulation. There are thus nine

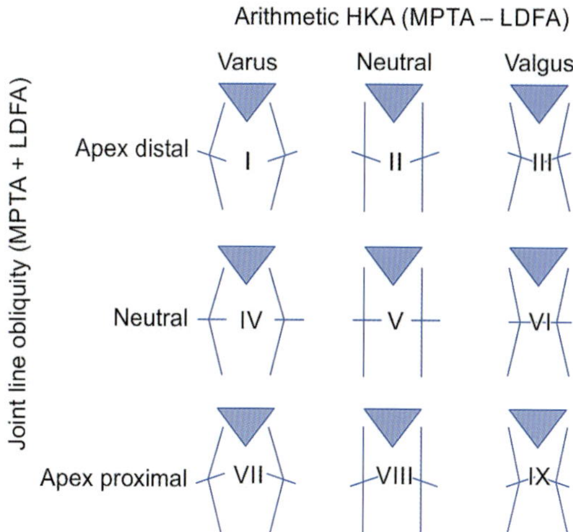

FIG. 3: Coronal plane alignment of the knee.

(HKA: hip-knee-ankle angle; mPTA: medial proximal tibial angle; LDFA: lateral distal femoral angle)

types of alignment, leading to different scenarios of overall knee varus, neutral, and valgus alignment. This classification helps in deciding the type and position of the alignment, and the appropriate correction needed during surgery to get "normal" alignment, or its maintenance in "kinematic" alignment post-total knee arthroplasty (TKA) **(Fig. 3)**.

"Normal" Rotational Alignment

As the proximal tibial cut is performed perpendicular to the mechanical tibial axis, instead of the anatomically correct 3° varus, to obtain a rectangular flexion gap, the femoral component must be rotated externally 3° (and the cut made in 3° external rotation with respect to the posterior femoral condylar axis) **(Fig. 4)**. However, the amount of rotation needed to rectangularize the flexion gap and/or equalize the flexion-extension gaps depend on the severity and type of preexisting "individual" alignment and the soft tissue balance restored. *This can therefore vary from 3° internal rotation to 9° external rotation.*

Patellofemoral Alignment

Patellofemoral stability is maintained by a combination of articular surface geometry and soft tissue restraints. Limbs with large Q-angle

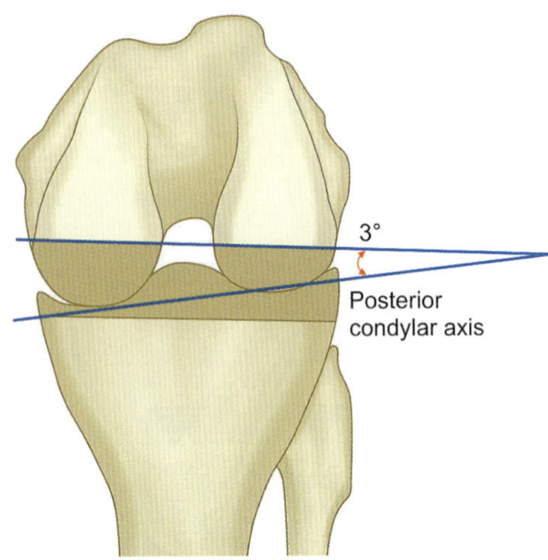

FIG. 4: External rotation of femur on tibia rectangularizes flexion gap.

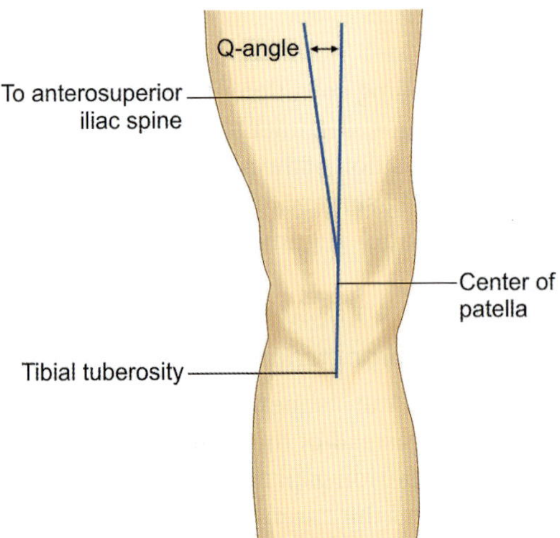

FIG. 5: Q-angle.

(angle between extended anatomical axis of femur, and line between center of patella and tibial tubercle) have a greater tendency to lateral patellar subluxation. The normal Q-angles are 14° in males, and 17° in females. Patella tracking depends on an interplay between the implant design and restoration of the appropriate femoral rotation, so as to avoid patella tilts/angulation, and negate the pull of large Q-angles **(Fig. 5)**.

KNEES WITH THE TOTAL KNEE ARTHROPLASTY PROSTHESIS (OPERATED KNEES)

The aim of TKA is to *either* reproduce anatomy or recreate as close as possible the individual "normal" biomechanical axis and kinematics of the limb. Implant systems designed for TKA follow one of the following principles:

- *Anatomically aligned TKA:* Recreation of the *normal* human mechanical and anatomical axes (most commonly, tibia in varus, femur in valgus, with overall slight limb varus). These are called *anatomically aligned* TKA designs (e.g., NK-II, Conformis knee).
- *Mechanically aligned TKA*: Production of a knee joint line *perpendicular* to the mechanical axis of both the femur, tibia, and an eventual HKA which is perpendicular to the ground in single/double-legged stance, called *mechanically aligned* TKA designs (e.g., PFC Sigma, NexGen).
- *Kinematically aligned (individually aligned) TKA*: Small *variations* of the above to produce any one of the *near-normal* axes (viz., "adjusted" mechanical axis, "adjusted" anatomical axis, "reverse" mechanical axis design, and "reverse" anatomical axis), the so-called *individualized alignment TKA* designs (usually used in conjunction with robotic-assisted TKA).

Tibial components are generally implanted perpendicular to the mechanical axis of the tibia, with posterior tilt dictated by the

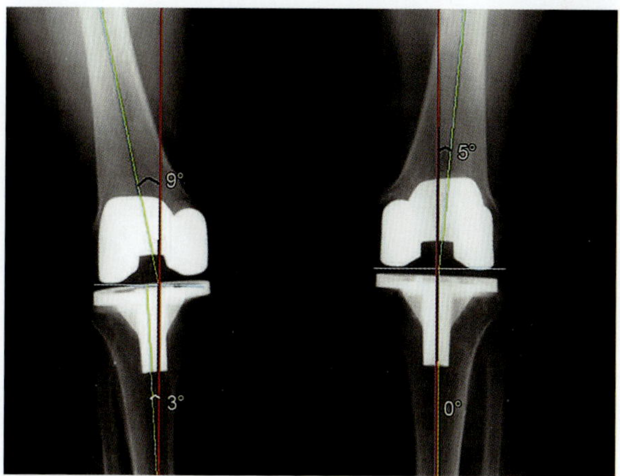

FIG. 6: Axes reconstruction with total knee arthroplasty (TKA) prosthesis (on radiography).

(Rt knee: kinematically aligned; Lt knee: mechanically aligned)

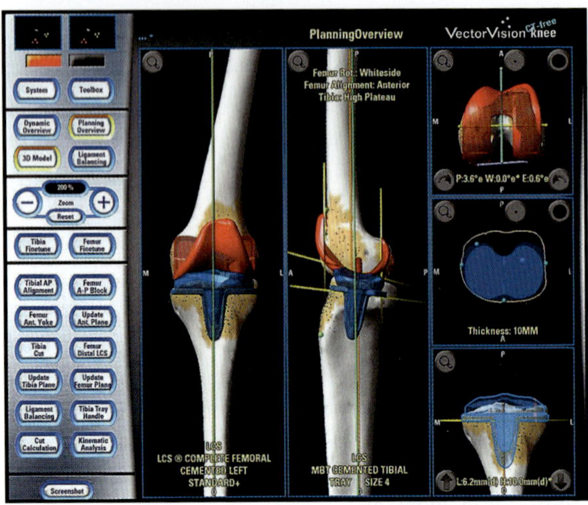

FIG. 7: Axes reconstruction with total knee arthroplasty (TKA) prosthesis (computer-assisted knee replacement).

flexion-extension gaps, whilst the femoral component is usually implanted in 5–6° valgus, the amount necessary to reestablish a neutral limb axis in "mechanical" alignment recreation. However, the components may be placed in slight varus (tibial and/or femoral components) or slight valgus (femoral and/or tibial component) to recreate the "kinematic", "reverse kinematic", or "individual" alignment, depending on the end-result desired **(Figs. 6 and 7)**.

Chapter 4

Getting Started: Implant Systems and Designs

A wide array of different implant systems and instrument designs are available today for total knee arthroplasty (TKA) surgery, the potential for the beginner to get confused and discouraged is immense. Classifying implants into fixed-bearing and mobile-bearing, and further into posterior cruciate ligament (PCL) substituting and retaining types resolves the confusion somewhat. *However, the advice to the novice is to stick with one design for the first few 100 cases, as all designs will then seem to have a set pattern.*

To this effect, we present the most commonly and widely used system for understanding, viz., the Attune knee (DePuy Synthes).

The components include the femoral implant (right and left, PCL substituting or retaining, and sizes 1, 2, 3, 3N, 4, 4N, 5, 5N, 6 and 7), the tibial tray (universal for right and left, sizes matching femoral components), the patellar button (eccentric, dome-shaped, and 3-pegged), and the Attune tibial insert (with post-and-cam mechanism) **(Fig. 1)**.

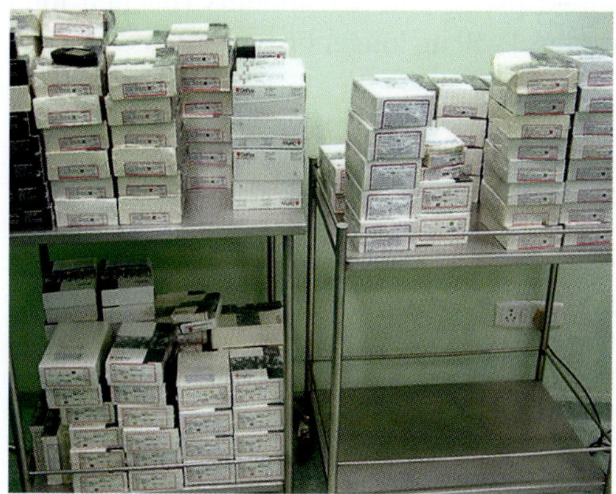

FIG. 1: Total knee arthroplasty (TKA) implants (inventory).

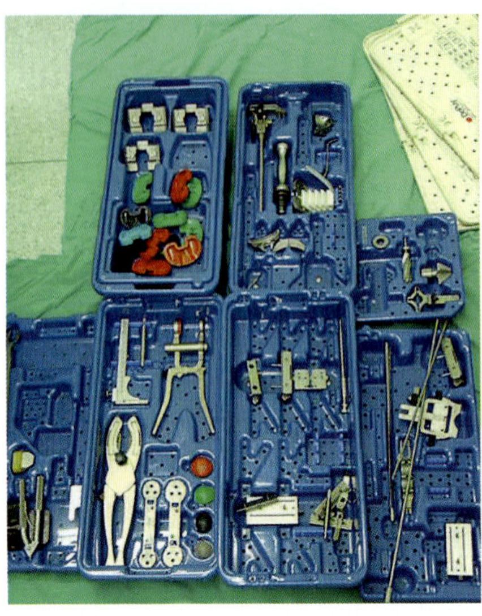

FIG. 2: Total knee arthroplasty (TKA) instrumentation sets.

The instrumentation involved include the intramedullary rod and jigs for the femur (for distal, anteroposterior, notch and chamfer cuts), the intra- and extramedullary rod and jigs for the tibial baseplate, with the keel punch, and instruments for patellar resurfacing **(Fig. 2)**.

With advent of computer-assisted, robotic-assisted, and 3D printed instruments and implants for TKA, the inventory needed in the operation theater (OT) is reduced, as is the need for additional sizes of implants (falling out of the range of the sizes as decided by the preoperative plan), and instruments (needed for mechanical alignment surgery) will no longer be necessary.

Chapter 5

Surgical Approaches

The standard surgical approach used in a majority of total knee arthroplasty (TKA) surgery is the medial parapatellar approach (used in >90% cases). The knee can be approached surgically in the ways given in the following text.

MEDIAL PARAPATELLAR APPROACH

Standard skin midline incision, deep approach through the interval between the vastus intermedius and vastus medialis, maintaining a thick medial skin flap. This retinacular incision is usually extended proximally along the length of the quadriceps tendon (leaving a 3–4 mm cuff of tendon on the vastus medialis for later closure), continued around the medial side of the patella, and extending distally to about 3–4 cm onto the anteromedial tibial surface (along the medial border of the patellar tendon). Thereafter, subperiosteal stripping of the anteromedial capsule and deep medial collateral ligament (MCL) is conducted off the tibia (depending on the release needed, to the posteromedial corner of the knee) **(Figs. 1 and 2)**.

This standard approach is recommended in all varus deformities, and mild valgus and flexion deformities **(Figs. 3 and 4)**. It is also the preferred approach in most revision TKA surgeries.

Other Medial Approaches

Subvastus

The subvastus "Southern" approach, advocated by Hoffman, Plaster, and Murdock, is different from the standard approach, in that the skin incision is slightly medial to the midline, and carried deeper below the vastus medialis (as the name implies). The proximal retinacular

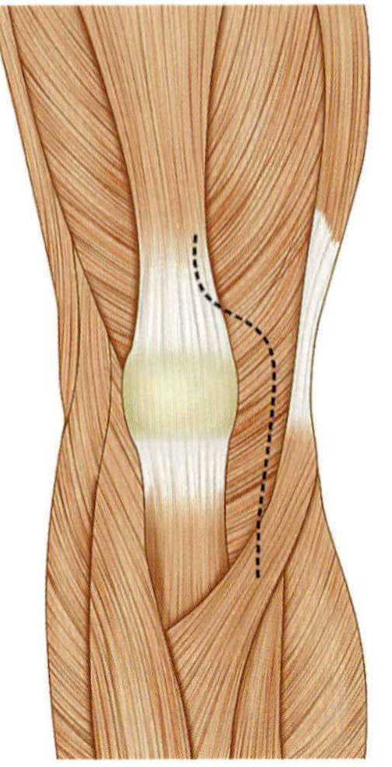

FIG. 1: Standard (medial parapatellar) approach: Superficial dissection.

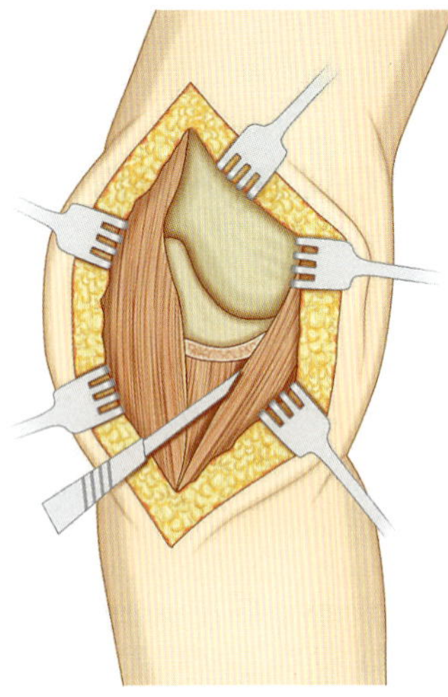

FIG. 2: Standard (medial parapatellar) approach: Deep dissection.

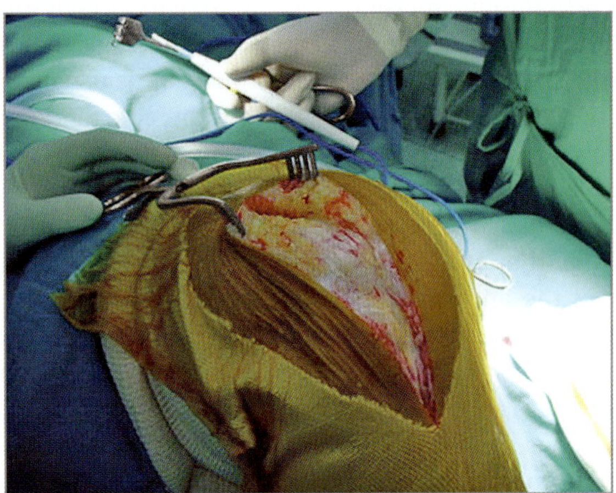

FIG. 3: Standard (medial parapatellar) approach: Superficial dissection (clinical picture).

incision involves incising the superficial fascia overlying the vastus medialis and bluntly mobilizing the distal medial border of the vastus medialis all the way to the medial intermuscular septum.

This extensor mechanism sleeve is then subluxated laterally for exposure.

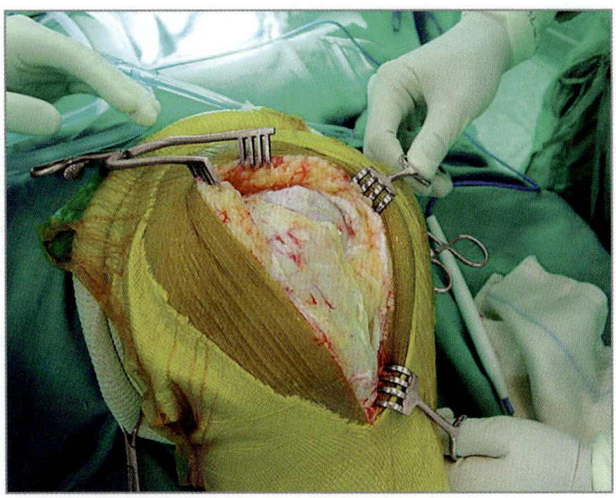

FIG. 4: Standard (medial parapatellar) approach: Deep dissection (clinical picture).

Leaving the extensor mechanism intact results in a more rapid return of quadriceps strength, preserving more patella vascularity, improving patient satisfaction while decreasing postoperative pain, and a reduced need for lateral release. However, exposure is sometimes limited and can be a problem (specially in obese patients and those with previous knee procedures).

Midvastus

The midvastus approach, described by Engh and Parks, also resembles the standard approach; however, the deeper plane passes obliquely through (and thus splitting) the vastus medialis muscle. It thus also differs from the subvastus approach (vastus medialis muscle is split in line with its fibers rather than subluxated laterally in its entirety). This split starts at the superomedial border of the patella (extending proximally and medially, toward the intermuscular septum).

These (subvastus and midvastus) approaches preserve the superior genicular artery (to the patella and quadriceps tendon). Obesity, previous upper tibial osteotomy, and limited preoperative flexion of <80° are relative contraindications **(Figs. 5A to D)**.

Therefore, these approaches have been recommended for moderately unstable, nonobese, nonfixed varus and valgus knees. *A mini version of the midvastus approach is the standard approach for medial unicompartment knee arthroplasty (UKA).*

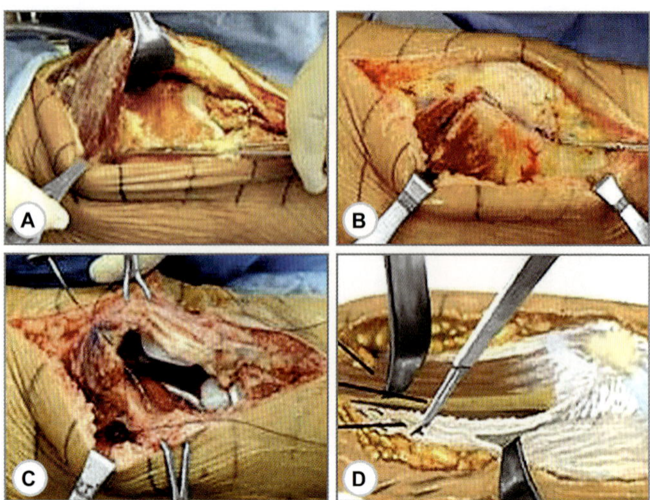

FIGS. 5A TO D: Alternative surgical approaches: (A) Subvastus approach; (B) Midvastus approach; (C) Lateral approach; and (D) Z-lengthening of lateral structures in lateral approach.

Lateral Approach

A midline (or slightly lateral to the midline) skin incision, with the deeper plane going through the lateral retinaculum bordering the patella (lateral parapatellar retinacular incision) has been advocated by Keblish et al. in patients with valgus knees. Deeper dissection is through the space between the vastus intermedius and vastus lateralis. Others have combined this approach with a tibial tubercle osteotomy to improve exposure and relax extensor mechanism tension.

Advantages include improved patellofemoral tracking and increased visibility of the lateral structures (more so in valgus knees needing sequential releasing for ligamentous balancing), as well as an ability to gradually titrate the releases needed to balance a valgus arthritic knee **(Fig. 6)**.

The lateral approach is recommended for fixed valgus knees (with associated lateral patellar subluxation and/or significant rotation).

Revision Approaches

Whenever possible, one should use the previous skin incision (when two previous incisions already exist, the more lateral of the two

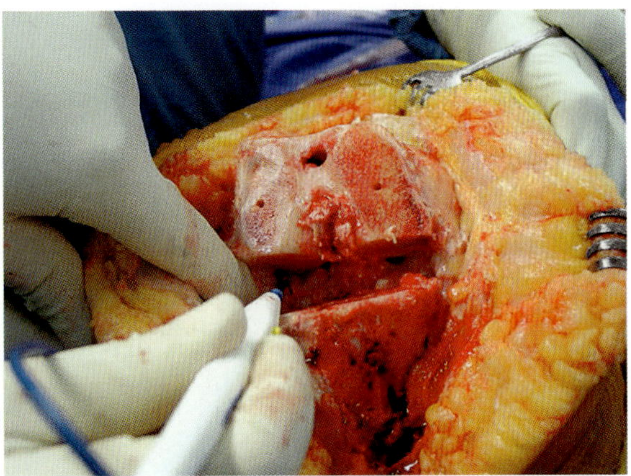

FIG. 6: Lateral approach: Precrust lengthening of posterolateral structures.

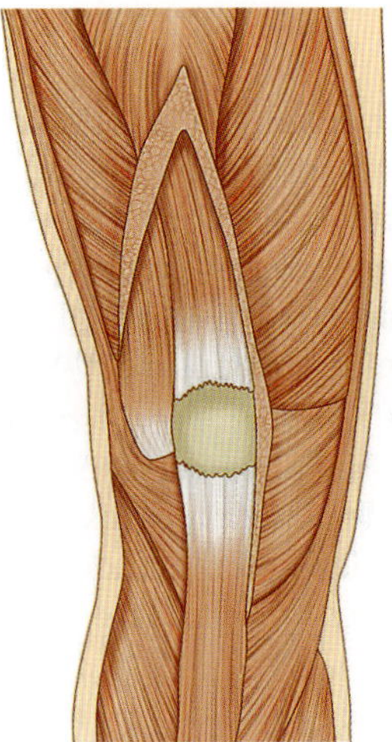

FIG. 7: Quadriceps "V-Y" plasty.

should be selected, if possible, because of more favorable medial superficial blood supply).

The medial parapatellar is usually the workhorse when it comes to revision TKA. Sometimes, however, an additional exposure method (one of, or a combination of, those discussed in the following text) may be needed.

- *Quadriceps turndown procedure (modified by Scott and Siliski) and Quadriceps V-Y plasty* **(Fig. 7)**: Standard medial parapatellar

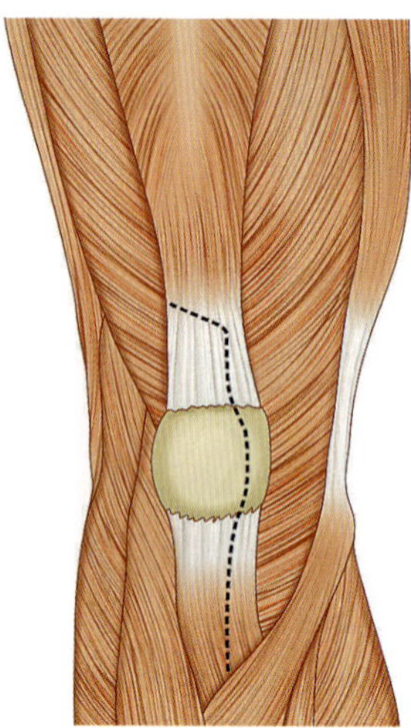

FIG. 8: The "rectus snip" procedure.

retinacular deep incision, with an additional limb extending as an "inverted V" across the quadriceps tendon through the lateral patellar retinaculum, as distal as needed. During closure, this inverted "V" can be converted to a "Y" (by allowing the patella and attached quadriceps tendon to be advanced distally), permitting lengthening and closure (V-Y quadricepsplasty).

- *The rectus "snip" (Insall's modification of the quadriceps turndown)* **(Fig. 8)**: The proximal extent of a medial parapatellar arthrotomy is extended laterally across the quadriceps tendon to incise the rectus tendon and the underlying tendinous insertion of the vastus muscles (to facilitate knee flexion and patella subluxation/eversion).
- *Tibial tubercle osteotomy (modified by Whiteside and Ohl)* **(Fig. 9)**: An 8–10 cm segment of bone (which includes the tibial tubercle and a portion of the anterior crest of the tibia distal to it) is osteotomized and reflected laterally (while maintaining vascularity to this fragment through the laterally attached anterior compartment musculature).

Barrack et al. compared the standard medial arthrotomy, rectus snip, V-Y quadricepsplasty, and tibial tubercle osteotomy in revision TKA. The outcomes with the standard approach and rectus snip were identical in all clinical parameters.

V-Y quadricepsplasty resulted in greater extensor lag but increased patient satisfaction compared with tibial tubercle osteotomy, which

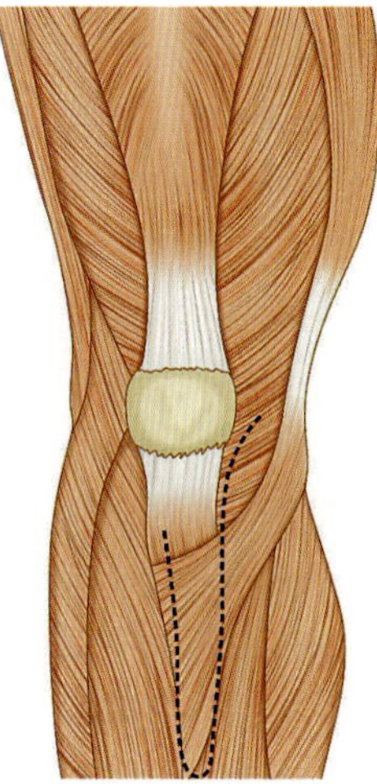

FIG. 9: The "tibial tubercle" osteotomy.

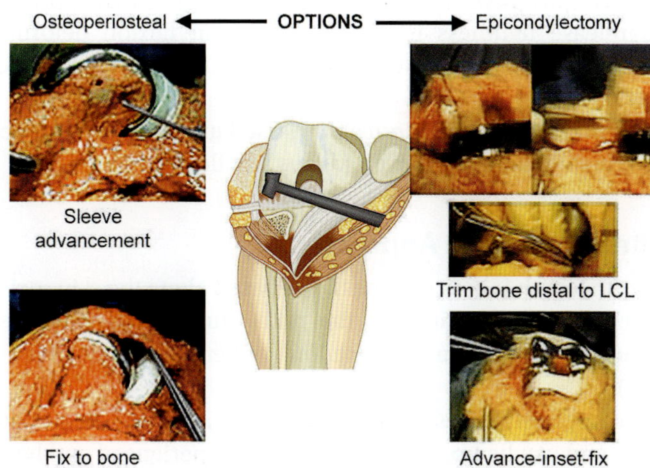

FIG. 10: Extended approach option: Osteoperiosteal sleeve advancement and medial epicondylectomy.

(LCL: lateral collateral ligament)

resulted in more difficulty with kneeling and stooping. Both the quadricepsplasty and osteotomy groups had significantly lower outcome ratings compared with the standard arthrotomy and rectus snip **(Fig. 10)**.

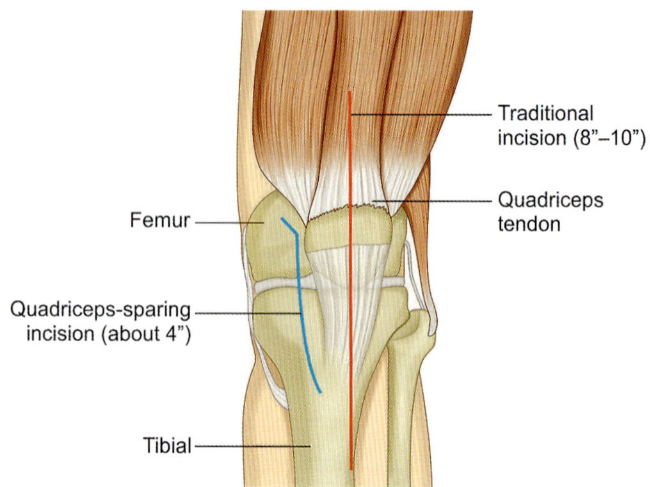

FIG. 11: The minimally invasive incision vis-à-vis standard incision.

- *Medial epicondyle slide osteotomy:* Used in extended approaches to release tightness in severe varus and flexion deformities (wherein a sliding osteotomy of the medial epicondyle is performed).
- *Lateral epicondyle slide osteotomy:* Used in extended approaches to release tightness in severe valgus and flexion deformities.

Minimally Invasive Approaches

Shorter in length (about 4 inches), it is based along the skin incision and deep dissection lines of the midvastus/medial parapatellar approaches, with lateral subluxation (rather than eversion of the patella).

It completely preserves quadriceps integrity and patella stability and can be used as one gets more experienced and has the appropriate instrumentation **(Fig. 11)**.

Chapter 6

Indications and Contraindications

INDICATIONS

Total knee arthroplasty (TKA) surgery is indicated in advanced osteoarthritis—either primary (usually a polyarticular degenerative arthritis of unknown origin, occurring after the age of 45 years), or secondary (usually monoarticular, following a prolonged reaction of a joint to mechanical derangement, pyogenic infection, congenital anomaly, physeal separation, ligamentous instability, or intra-articular fracture producing articular surface incongruity, common in obese patients >50 years of age), clinically manifested as unremitting or unresolving pain in the affected knee joint (with or without associated swelling and deformity) **(Fig. 1)**. Often, a

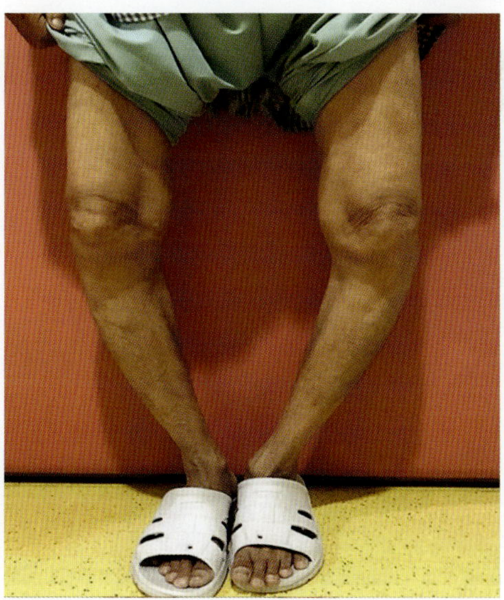

FIG. 1: Clinical picture of typical patient needing total knee arthroplasty (TKA).

sufficient trial of conservative treatment has been offered, and the patient has either not responded well enough, or the complaints persist/accentuate.

The primary aim of TKA surgery is to relieve pain (caused by the advanced arthritis), usually with deformity correction, and is commonly recommended in the older sedentary patient; and occasionally in younger patients with limited function (due to systemic inflammatory arthritis with multiple joint involvement). Severe pain arising due to joint destruction following chondrocalcinosis and/or gout/pseudogout is an occasional indication. Other pathological conditions that may necessitate TKA include post-traumatic and postinfective arthritis.

Radiographs in such patients typically show a severe reduction in joint space [medial and/or lateral, with osteophyte formation, development of angular deformity (varus/valgus)], with occasional subluxation of the tibia. Depending on the severity of the wear and tear, there may additionally be bone defects seen on the plain X-rays **(Fig. 2)**.

The following have been defined as extended indications:

- Fractures around arthritic joints
- Unstable knees (post-traumatic)
- Revision of failed unicompartment knee arthroplasty (UKA) **(Fig. 3)**
- Fused knees

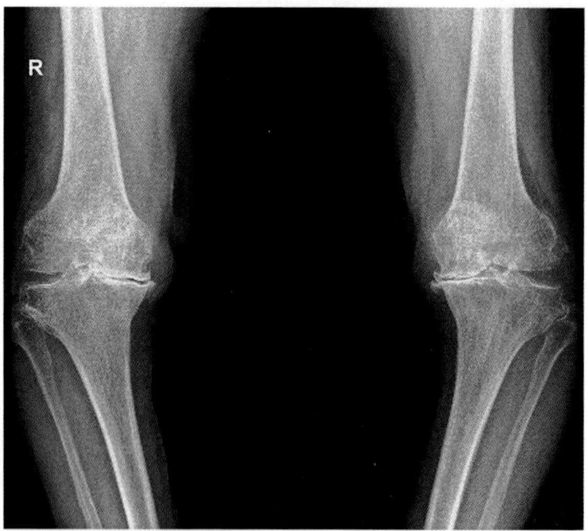

FIG. 2: Typical X-rays of patient needing total knee arthroplasty (TKA).

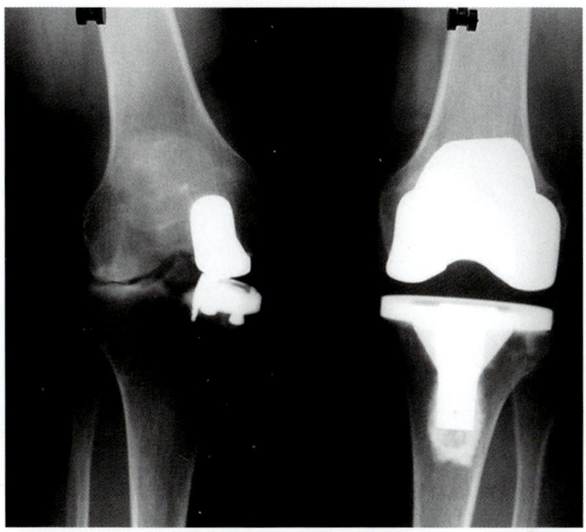

FIG. 3: Extended indications for knee replacement: Failed unicompartment knee replacement.

Deformity can become the principal indication for TKA in patients with moderate arthritis and variable levels of pain (when the progression of deformity begins to limit or threaten the expected positive outcomes of surgery).

CONTRAINDICATIONS

Absolute contraindications include recent or current knee *sepsis*, or a remote source of ongoing infection. Extensor mechanism discontinuity or severe dysfunction, recurvatum deformity secondary to muscular weakness, isolated deformity/limb length discrepancy without pain, Charcot's (neuropathic) joints **(Fig. 4)**, and the presence of a painless, well-functioning knee arthrodesis were also once considered absolute contraindications but are now amenable to treatment using hinged knee implants (albeit with limited longevity).

Relative contraindications include all medical conditions that compromise the patient's ability to withstand anesthesia, the metabolic demands of surgery and/or wound healing [including significant atherosclerotic disease of the operative leg, unfavorable skin conditions (such as psoriasis) within the operative field, morbid obesity, recurrent urinary tract infections, and a history of

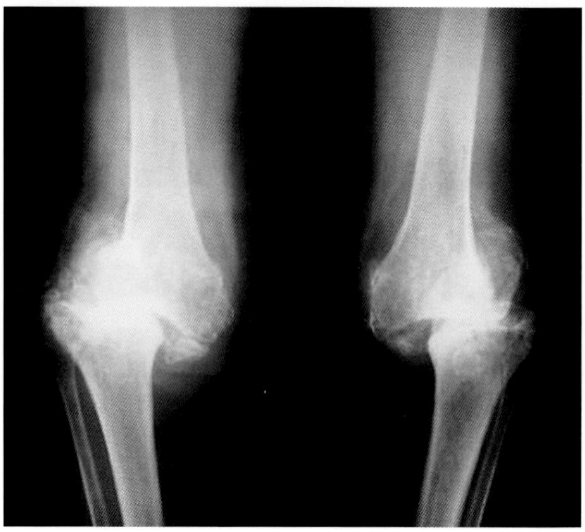

FIG. 4: Contraindication for knee replacement: Charcot's joints.

osteomyelitis in the proximity of the knee], as well as the significant rehabilitation necessary to ensure a favorable functional outcome.

It must never be forgotten that we are there to *treat the patient, and not the X-rays.*

Chapter 7

Preoperative Preparation

Preoperatively, it is imperative that the surgeon and his team familiarize themselves with the operating theater, implant systems, and equipment. Preoperative preparation can thus be tackled under the following heads.

INVENTORY CHECK

Detailed inventory of equipment needed for the surgery is essential (including the tourniquet, suction apparatus, and diathermy machines, as well as sufficient drapes, towels, and surgical gowns). A dry run before the D-day brings to the fore many small requirements that are usually taken for granted, the ready availability of which reduces surgical time, whilst also minimizing complications.

General and specialized orthopedic instruments, adequate arrangement for sterilization, and basic sets (needed for management of complications, if any) should be ready and available at hand.

With the advent of computer-assisted and robotic-assisted total knee arthroplasty (TKA), other sterilizing drapes as well as disposables and spare parts (including tracking balls/spheres, batteries, etc.) should be arranged beforehand.

OPERATION THEATER REQUIREMENTS

Laminar air flow systems facilitating sterile operating environments, minimal traffic of personnel, strict aseptic and safe techniques, maintenance of adequate environmental parameters (temperature, humidity, and ventilation), and trained and coordinated staff are essential prerequisites to a good outcome. Adequate lighting and

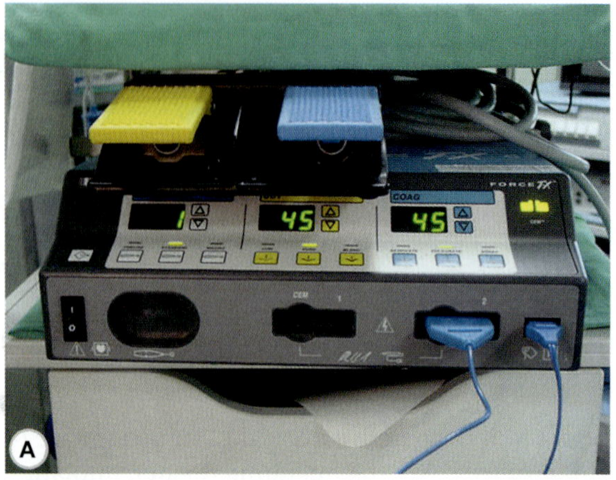

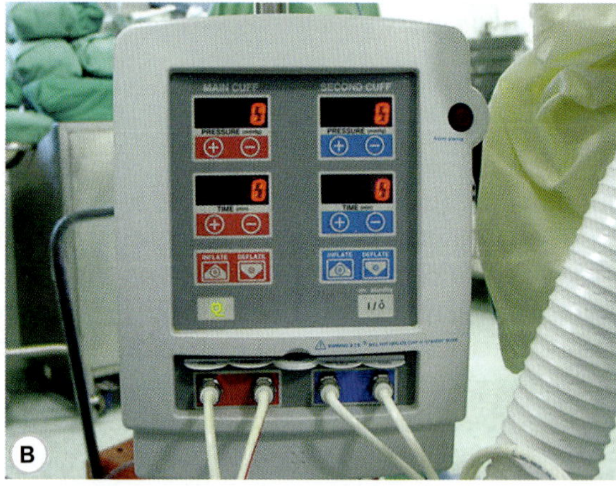

FIGS. 1A AND B: (A) Diathermy apparatus; (B) Electronic tourniquet.

properly functioning electronic equipment further facilitate a stress-free surgery **(Figs. 1 to 4)**.

A useful checklist to be followed includes:

- Train and synchronize the operation theater (OT) staff available to work under the team leader.
- Operating room to be sterilized overnight.
- Check instrumentation set inventory (and autoclave them).
- Check implant component inventory.

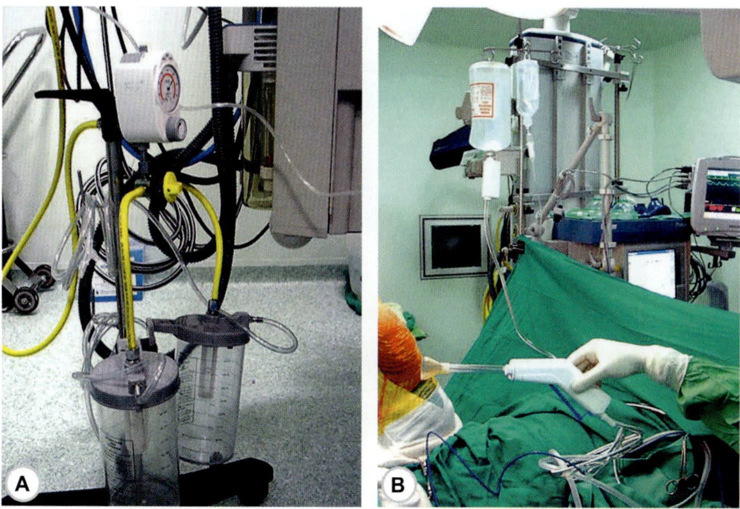

FIGS. 2A AND B: (A) Suction apparatus; (B) Pulsatile lavage system.

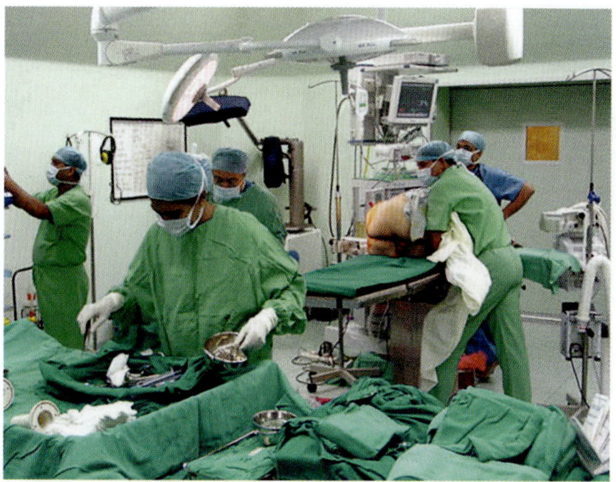

FIG. 3: Good operation theater (OT) environment.

- Keep extra bone cement packets.
- Keep fracture fixation sets (small and large fragment) as well as implants (plates/screws) on standby.
- Ensure a functioning image intensifier/C-arm.

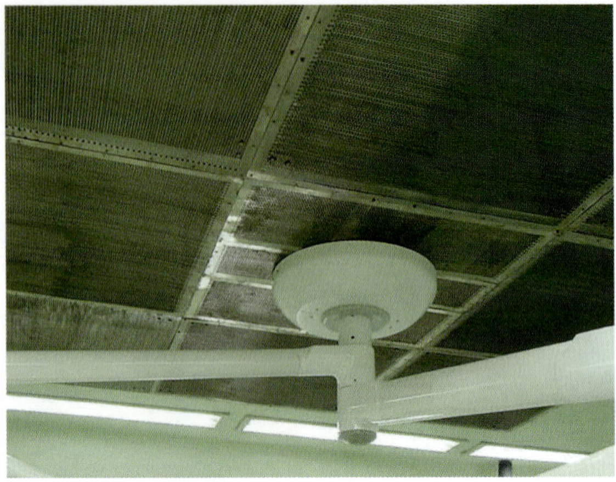

FIG. 4: Laminar air flow system.

Chapter 8

Preoperative Clinical Assessment

Total knee arthroplasty (TKA) surgery is a planned event. Planning the patient's progress through a good preoperative assessment, well-executed surgery, and good postoperative rehabilitation is therefore essential.

A thorough patient assessment (to gauge medical/surgical fitness, as well as psychological readiness) prior to surgery helps in ruling out unnecessary and unsuccessful surgery. Detailed history taking and a thorough physical examination help identify the need for surgery, and physical and mental fitness (for both anesthesia and surgical procedure is essential, with particular attention to the local skin condition, limb vascularity, and neuromuscular capability, viz., limb sensations, quadriceps/hamstring power). Further, an adequate risk factor assessment [with special reference to deep vein thrombosis (DVT), infection, anesthesia risk, and stress tolerance] as well as understanding of current medication; needs to be properly documented, evaluated, and appropriate specialist clearance taken. With the advent of accelerated physiotherapy rehab programs, it is also good to get the patient prepped for the physiotherapy regimen that he/she will need (prehabilitation), ensuring optimized local parameters before the actual surgery.

BEFORE ADMISSION

- The patient is preferably admitted a day prior to the surgery, an attempt already having been made to rule out any infective focus (with preoperative assessment and investigations).
- Detailed history taking must include any local procedure done and/or any complication in the past. *Special emphasis must be placed on any history of varicose ulcers, DVT, or pulmonary embolism (PE).*

- The adjoining hip and ankle joints must be evaluated in detail for fixed deformities.
- Quadriceps/Hamstring muscle strength will determine post-operative rehabilitation and must be recorded. Strength in upper limbs is noted where the patient has a polyarticular disease (inflammatory arthropathies). Current ambulatory status is noted.
- Preanesthetic check-up is completed. Multidisciplinary approach for surgical fitness is sought (internist, cardiologist, diabetologist, nephrologist, etc.), where needed.
- Blood/blood products need to be arranged where indicated, preoperative transfusion is avoided.
- Anticoagulants, antiplatelet aggregatory drugs, and nonsteroidal anti-inflammatory drugs (NSAIDs) are stopped 2–4 days prior to surgery, disease modifying rheumatic drugs (DMRDs) can be withheld for a week before surgery and recommenced 2 weeks after the surgery (wound healing issues).

PREOPERATIVE JOINT ASSESSMENT

- The joint(s) to be operated upon is (are) identified, especially in patients with polyarticular involvement. The more painful side is recorded, as it should be operated upon *first* in bilateral joint involvement, where simultaneous surgery is planned. Local skin condition/any previous operative scar is noted.
- Pain scoring, knee scoring, and range of motion are recorded **(Fig. 1)**.

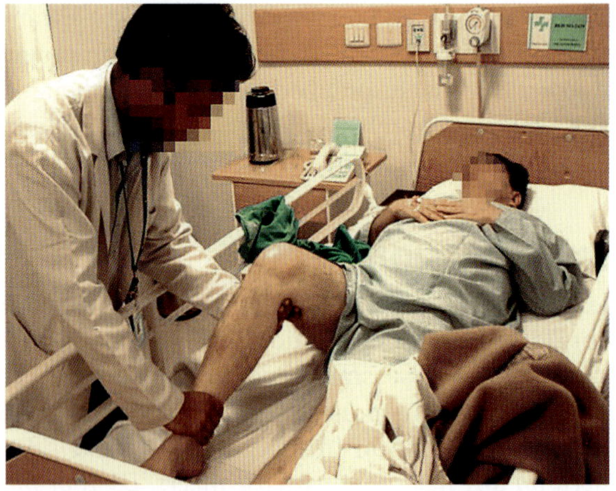

FIG. 1: Clinical evaluation of patient.

INFORMED CONSENT

- Valid written informed consent, mentioning the diagnosis, the side to be operated (left/right/both), including the phrase "*advised* not to squat or sit cross-legged on the ground after the surgery", explained to the patient in a language that he/she understands, and recorded as such **(Fig. 2)**.
- *Inform the patient of the likely complications:* Infection, DVT, PE, and anesthetic risks, as appropriate. Include the possibility of additional/modifying procedures (need for occult/iatrogenic fracture fixation, stem extenders where anticipated, bone grafting of defects where indicated, etc.).
- Patient should sign on the dotted line and a witness, a close relative, to countersign on the same paper. High-risk consent is taken where relevant.

EVENING BEFORE AND MORNING OF SURGERY

- Overnight fasting and early morning wash. Avoid shaving the part before surgery, paint the limb (groin to toes) with betadine, and drape with sterile sheets, check and mark the operated side (if unilateral). This step may be done away with in high volume or dedicated orthopedic and sports medicine centers.
- Morning medicines with a sip of water. Standby cardiologist/ intensive care unit (ICU), etc., are prepared, if need be. The patient is then shifted to the operation theater (OT) with relevant X-rays.

IN THE OPERATION THEATER

- Supine position, shave/trim the part that is expected to be in the operative site, put a sandbag under the hip (if unilateral). Tourniquet (if used) must be applied over upper thigh **(Fig. 3)**.
- Scrubbing with ioprep/betascrub/savlon, followed by painting of the leg from groin to toes with three layers of betadine, and then cutasept/sterillium. The leg is draped free in a stockinet, after routine draping. Strict adherence to *no-touch principle* **(Fig. 4)**.

Injectable [intravenous (IV)] prophylactic antibiotics, after test dose, just before the tourniquet is inflated (if used), or just before the incision (if not used).

INFORMED CONSENT FOR TOTAL KNEE REPLACEMENT

Date of Admission: ____________

MEDICAL CONDITION AND PROCEDURE (to be filled by the patient or the Doctor to document in patient's own words)

The doctor has explained that I/my patient have/has the following medical condition: ....

I/my patient have/has been advised to undergo the following treatment/ procedure as explained: ....

....

See patient information sheet – "Total Knee Replacement (TKR)" for more details

Procedure: The orthopaedic surgeon will remove the damaged cartilage and bone and then position the new metal and plastic joint surfaces to restore the alignment and function of the knee

Anaesthesia: Please see your **"Anaesthesia Consent Form"**. This gives you information of the General Risks of Surgery. If you have any concern(s), talk these over with your anaesthetist.

Risks of this Procedure & problems related to recovery:
While majority of patients have an uneventful surgery and recovery, few cases may be associated with complications. These are seen infrequently and not all the ones listed below are applicable to one individual. However it is important that you are aware of some of the common complications/risks that may arise out of this procedure and possible problems related to recovery which are as below:
Note: The listed risks and complications are not all inclusive. (Details of risks and complications are present in the "Patient Information Literature")

		Patient Specific risks:
(a) Clots in the legs	(i) Loss of blood supply to the leg	1)
(b) Wound infection	(j) Temperature disturbance to the operated leg	2)
(c) Dislocation of the knee joint	(k) Stiff knee joint	3)
(d) The bones around the joint may break	(l) Infection around the prosthesis years later	4)
(e) The kneecap may break	(m) Increased risks in obese and diabetic patients	
(f) The artificial joint will loosen or wear out	(n) Increased risk in smokers	
(g) Numbness by the cut		
(h) Numbness/ paralysis of the foot		

The benifits from the surgery may include increase in mobility, decrease in pain and improved quality of life.

I hereby authorize Dr.......... and those he may designate as associates or assistants according his/her stage of training/ability to perform upon me .... **Total Knee Replacement.**

Patient Consent:

- I have been provided with and explained the Patient Information Literature regarding the condition, treatment, procedure, risks and other associated information.
- I have been provided with and explained the Anaesthesia informed consent form.
- The doctor has explained my medical condition and proposed treatment/procedure. I have been explained and have understood the risks known to be attached with the planned treatment /procedure including the risks that are specific to me, and their likely outcomes.
- The doctor has explained other relevant/alternate treatment options and their associated risks. The doctor has also explained the risks of not having the procedure. I have understood the likelihood of success of the procedure. I have been given the choice to take a second opinion.
- I understand that the treatment/procedure may include blood/ blood products transfusion.

Continued overleaf

Patient Name:

Date:

Patients Signature:

Time:

Med/May 18/Ortho 472/Rev-1

FIG. 2: *Continued*

Continued

- I understand that if organs, limbs or tissues are removed during the surgery that these may be retained for tests and shall be disposed of sensitively by the hospital as per the regulatory provisions
- The doctor has explained and it has been agreed to me that if immediate life-threatening events occur during the treatment/procedure, they will be treated according to the prevalent medical norms.
- It has been explained to me, that during the course of or subsequent to the Operation/Procedure, unforeseen conditions may be revealed or encountered which may necessitate urgent surgical or other procedures in addition to or different from those contemplated. In such exigency, I further request and authorize the above named Physician / Surgeon or his designee to perform such additional surgical or other procedures as he or they consider necessary or desirable in my interest. I understand and agree that in such condition there will be no requirement of any additional consent from me or my family members/attendants.
- I declare that no guarantee of what so ever nature has been given by anyone as to the results that may be obtained.
- I consent to if any photographing or televising of the operation(s) or procedure(s) to be performed, including appropriate portions of my body, for medical, scientific or educational, and marketing purposes. However suitable precautions shall be taken by the hospital that my identity is not revealed anywhere. I have no objection to use of my medical records for research purposes without revealing any identity.
- For purposes of advancing medical education, I consent to the admittance of observers to the operating room.
- I understand that I have the right to refuse treatment or withdraw consent at any time. I agree that any such refusal/withdrawal shall be in writing and acknowledged by the Hospital. And I shall be solely responsible for the outcome of such refusal.
- I have been informed / explained about the likelihood of pain post treatment / procedure / examination and the options of pain management such as oral / intravenous / intramuscular / epidural / Patient-controlled analgesia (PCA) etc.

I certify that I have received complete information and fully understood the above consent statement, that all blanks requiring insertion or completion were filled in, prior to the time of my signature, and that this consent is given with stable mind, freely, voluntarily and without reservation.

Patient/Attendant to write the below line in his/her own handwriting if literate: "I certify that I have had the opportunity to ask questions regarding the ailment and procedure and they have been explained to me to my satisfaction in the language I understand." ....

....

....

....

Patient/Substitute Decision Maker	**Witness**	**Interpreter**
Reason for substitute decision maker	Name:	Interpreter used: Yes/No
Contact no. of substitute decision maker	Relationship:	Name:
Name:	Signature:	Translation given in:
Relationship:	Date & Time:	Signature:
Signature:	Contact no.:	Date & Time:
Date & Time:	Address:	Contact no.:

Doctor's Statement: I have explained the patient's condition, the procedure and the risks, likely consequences if those risks occur and the significant risks and problems specific to this patient. I have given the Patient/ Guardian an opportunity to ask questions about any of the above matters and raise any other concerns, which I have answered as fully as possible.
I am of the opinion that the Patient/ Substitute Decision Maker understood the above information

Name of Doctor:	Signature:
Designation:	Date & Time:

FIG. 2: Valid informed consent form (pages 1 and 2).

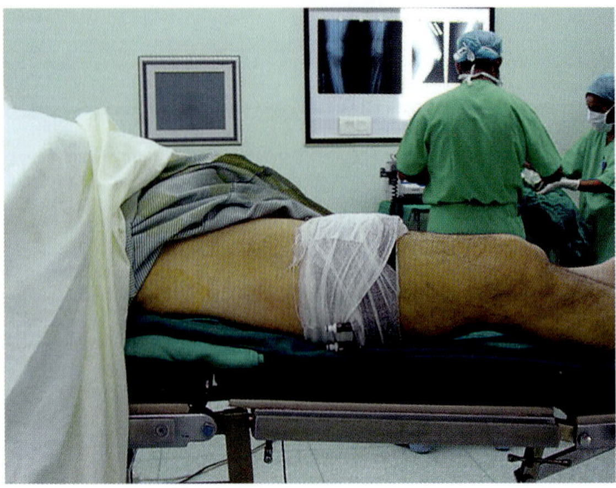

FIG. 3: Patient position and leg position in the operating theater.

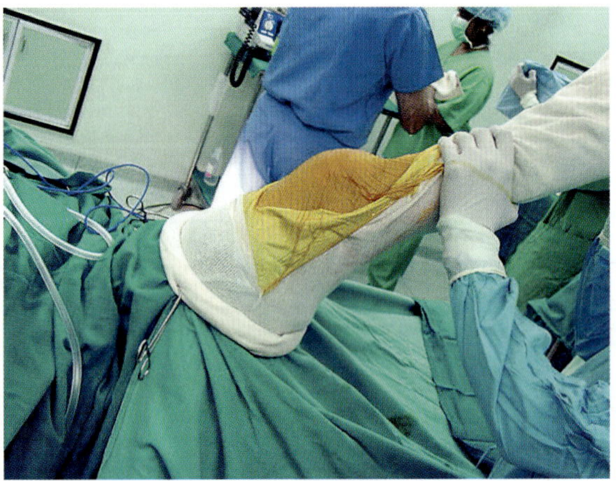

FIG. 4: Painted and draped extremity.

Chapter 9

Radiology and Templating

Radiological assessment is achieved with the *most recent* antero-posterior (AP) (standing), lateral, and skyline views routinely (and stress views, where needed). An assessment of the implant size, any bony defect, and stress fractures completes the relevant radiology **(Fig. 1)**.

Traditional method of templating involves getting true preoperative standing AP and lying lateral radiographs [alternatively, computed tomography (CT) tomographs] of the affected limbs. Tracings are made marking the anatomical and mechanical axes of the femora and tibiae. The altered mechanical axis of the limb is drawn and that desired is superimposed on it, so that cuts required to achieve the correct alignment are available preoperatively, thus guiding the angle and amount of cut needed in the proximal tibia, distal, and posterior femur. Assessment of size of the femoral, tibial, and patellar implants is also made and noted **(Figs. 2 and 3)**.

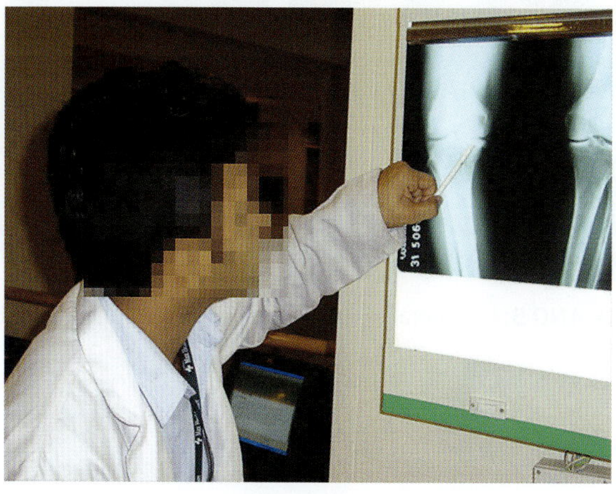

FIG. 1: Radiological evaluation of patient.

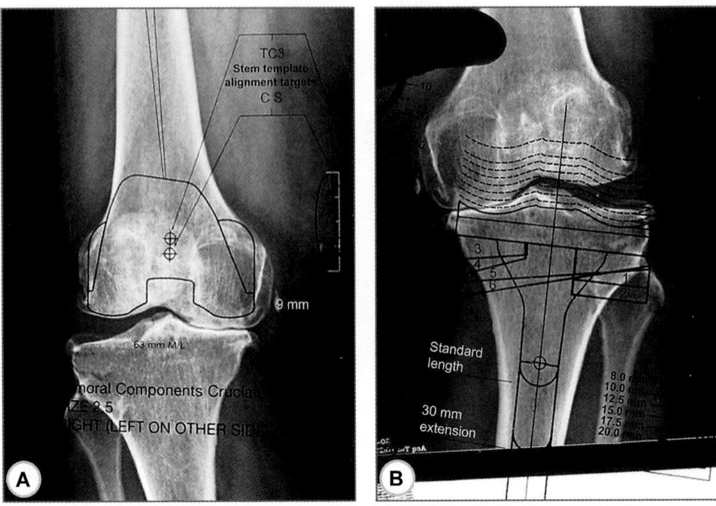

FIGS. 2A AND B: (A) Anteroposterior (AP) templating of femoral implant; and (B) tibial implant.

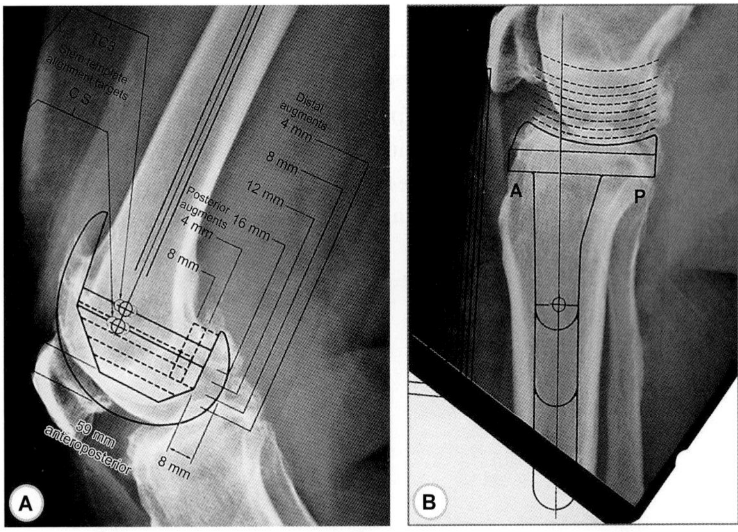

FIGS. 3A AND B: (A) Lateral templating of femoral implant; and (B) tibial implant.

Templating of preoperative X-rays is routinely performed before a total knee replacement. However, studies have revealed that traditional templating is highly subjective and observer dependent, with interobserver and intraobserver mismatch in 46.8% and 43.6% of readings, respectively, thus concluding that traditional preoperative templating is neither accurate nor reproducible. This system of templating for total knee arthroplasties is prone to error and can only be used as an approximate guide.

Currently, there are many digital software apps that help in templating, and this can therefore be done using even your mobile phone. Computer-assisted/robotic-assisted or 3D printed joints have inbuilt templating as part of their plan anyways.

Deformity, if any, is assessed and recorded in the sagittal plane (*flexion:* correctable/fixed), coronal plane (*varus/valgus:* correctable/fixed), and axially (rotation).

Chapter 10

Scoring

Knee scoring is essential to permit objective evaluation of the knee function (as well as of the patient as a whole) before and after surgery. A method of classification of patients and their outcome measures needs to be followed for adequate understanding of the results of knee replacement surgery. This then is the rationale behind scoring.

SYSTEMS

Many systems exist and have their own proponents, viz., hospital for special surgery (HSS) score, Oxford knee score (OKS), knee society score (KSS), to name a few.

We tend to follow the KSS, as it affords minimal inter- and intraobserver variability, and is relatively easy to document. This score involves the use of a simple multiple-choice questionnaire **(Fig. 1)** for the patient. The KSS has two components—the Pain Score and the Function Score.

Apart from this, there also exists a KSS roentgenographic score to evaluate postoperative radiographs of knee replacement patients.

KNEE SOCIETY SCORE

The KSS takes parameters such as pain, range of motion, stability, and the use of support while walking into account for calculation.

In 1989, the Knee Society published its revised knee rating system, so as to separate patients' overall functional ability from knee function alone. As a patient ages, the knee score may stay constant while functional ability declines because of factors unrelated to the status of the knee. To separate the two areas of function, the Knee Society *Clinical Rating System* has a separate knee score with 50 points

Knee Score

Patient Name____________________________________

Reg. No.________________ Age/Sex________________ DOA______________ DOP______________

Patient Reporting

Thank you for taking the time to help us better understand how your knee problem affects your daily life.

Please circle the answer that best describes your knee:

1. How much pain do you have when you are walking?
   - None
   - Mild or Occasional
   - Moderate
   - Severe
2. How much pain does your knee cause when going up and down stairs?
   - None
   - Mild or Occasional
   - Moderate
   - Severe
3. How much pain does your knee cause when you are at rest?
   - None
   - Mild or Occasional
   - Moderate
   - Severe
4. How does your knee affect your walking ability?
   - I can walk unlimited distances
   - I can walk 10–20 blocks
   - I can walk 5–10 blocks
   - I can walk 1–5 blocks
   - I can walk less than one blocks
   - I cannot walk at all
5. How do you go up stairs?
   - I go up stairs normally one foot infront of the other
   - I use the hand rail for balance
   - I use the hand rail to put myself up
   - I cannot climb stairs
6. How do you go down stairs?
   - I go down stairs normally one foot of the other
   - I use the hand rail for balance
   - I use the hand rail to support myself
   - I cannot come down stairs
7. How do you get out of a chair?
   - I get out of a chair normally without support
   - I use the arm rests for balance
   - I use the arm rests to push myself
   - I cannot get out of a chair
8. What type of support do you use when walkin?
   - None
   - Cane
   - 2 Canes
   - Walker

CLINICAL ASSESSMENT

9. Range of Motion
   - ....Degrees
10. Extension Lag
    - ....Degrees
11. Flexion Contracture
    - ....Degrees
12. Medial/Lateral Stability
    - 0–5 mm
    - 5–10 mm
    - >10 mm
13. Anterior/Posterior Stability
    - 0–5 mm
    - 5–10 mm
    - >10 mm
14. Alignment
    - ....Degrees

    Effusion (present/not)

    Joint Line Tenderness

FIG. 1: Knee society scoring (KSS) questionnaire.

Knee Findings		
Pain	**50 (Maximum)**	
Walking (insert the value associated with the result of question 1)		
None	35	
Mild or occasional	30	
Moderate	15	
Severe	0	
Stairs (Result of question 2)		
None	15	
Mild or occasional	10	
Moderate	5	
Severe	0	
ROM	**25 (Maximum)**	
(Result of question 9)		
50 = 1 point		
Stability	**25 (Maximum)**	
Medial/Lateral (Result of question 12)		
0–5 mm	15	
5–10 mm	10	
>10 mm	5	
Anterior/Posterior (Result of quesiton 13)		
0–5 mm	10	
5–10 mm	8	
>10 mm	5	
Deductions		
Extension lag (Result of question 10)		
None	0	
<4 degrees	–2	
5–10 degrees	–5	
>11 degrees	–10	
Flexion Contracture (Result of question 11)		
<5 degrees	0	
6–10	–3	
11–20 degrees	–5	
>20 degrees	–10	
Malalignment (Result of question 14)		
5–10 degrees	0	
(5°=–2 points)		
Pain at rest (Result of question 3)		
Mild	–5	
Moderate	–10	
Severe	–15	
Symptomatic plus objective	–0	
(Now, simply total the scores of each of these questions to obtain the total Knee Score of the patient)		
Knee Score	100 (Maximum) =	
Function Findings		
Walking (Result of question 4)		
Unlimited	55	
10–20 blocks	50	
5–10 blocks	35	
1–5 blocks	25	
<1 block	15	
Cannot	0	
Stairs Up (Result of quesiton 5)		
Normal	15	
Hands balance	12	
Hands pull	5	
Cannot or bizarre		
Stairs Down (Result of quesiton 6)		
Normal	15	
Hands balance	12	
Hands hold	5	
Cannot or bizarre	0	
Chair (Result of question 7)		
Normal	15	
Hands balance	12	
Hands pull	5	
Cannot	0	
Functional Deductions (Result of question 8)		
Cane	–2	
Crutches	–10	
Walker	–10	
Functional Score	100 (Maximum) =	

FIG. 2: Knee society pain and functional scoring chart.

for pain, 25 points for range of motion, and 25 points for stability. Points are deducted for flexion contracture, extension lag, and malalignment. A separate *Patient Function Score* assigns 50 points for stair climbing and 50 points for walking distance, with deductions for the use of walking aids **(Fig. 2)**.

Also in 1989, the Knee Society introduced the Total Knee Arthroplasty Roentgenographic Evaluation and Scoring System to standardize the roentgenographic parameters to be measured when reporting roentgenographic outcomes of total knee arthroplasty (TKA), which included an objective measurement of the component alignment, tibial surface coverage, presence of radiolucency, and a patellar problem list (that included angle of the prosthesis, eccentric component placement, subluxation, and dislocation) **(Fig. 3)**. A score is calculated for each component based on the width and extent of its associated radiolucencies. For a seven-zone tibial component, a nonprogressive score of 4 or less is probably insignificant, a score of

TKA Scoring System

Evaluator name ______ Date ______
Patient name/number ______ Preop ☐ Postop ☐
Surgeon name ______ Hospital number ______
X-ray date ______ Prior implants ______
Joint: Left knee ☐ Right knee ☐
Alignment: Recumbent ☐ Standing ☐

Anteroposterior — Angle in degrees
Femoral flexion (α) ______
Tibial angle (β) ______
Total valgus angle (Ω) ______
18" Film ______
3' Film ______

Lateral — Angle in degrees
Femoral flexion (γ) ± ______
Tibial angle (σ) ______

Implant/bone surface area
Percent area of tibial surface covered by implant

Radiolucencies: Indicate depth in millimeters in each zone

RLL 1 ___ 2 ___ 3 ___ 4 ___ 5 ___ 6 ___ 7 ___ Total ______

med. lat. RLL 1 ___ 2 ___ 3 ___ 4 ___ 5 ___ 6 ___ 7 ___ Total ______

ant. post. RLL 1 ___ 2 ___ 3 ___ Total ______

med. lat. ☐ OR ☐ RLL 1 ___ 2 ___ 3 ___ 4 ___ 5 ___ Total ______

Patellar problem list
Angle of prosthesis ______ Subluxation ______
Placement Med-Lat ______
Sup-Inf ______ Dislocation ______

FIG. 3: Knee society radiological scoring chart.

5–9 indicates a need for close follow-up for progression, and a score of 10 or more signifies possible or impending failure regardless of symptoms.

Preoperatively, the knee is scored according to the Knee Society Pain and Function scores. Patients are handed a multiple-choice questionnaire, followed by examination of the deformity and laxity. These are then fed into the database for reference and comparison with postoperative values.

Chapter 11

Surgical Technique: Standard Knee

PATIENT POSITIONING, INCISION, AND APPROACH

Position: Supine with rolled towel/sandbag under ipsilateral hip **(Fig. 1)**.

Skin incision: Midline or slightly lateral paramidline (lower mid-thigh to tibial tubercle).

Deep incision and approach: Medial parapatellar approach **(Fig. 2)**.

Placement of Hohman's retractors: Lateral tibial, medial tibial, and posterior tibial **(Fig. 3)**.

Structures cut and removed: Menisci (medial and lateral), ligaments [anterior cruciate ligament (ACL) posterior cruciate ligament

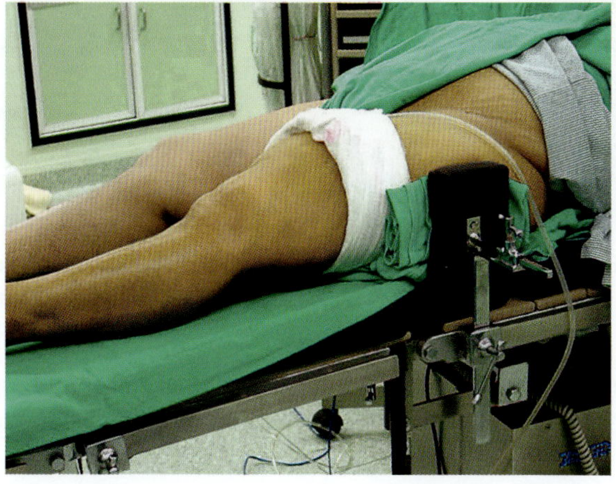

FIG. 1: Supine position with side support with tourniquet.

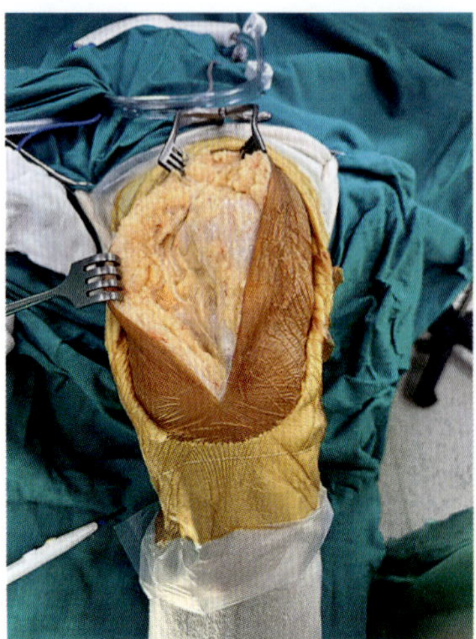

FIG. 2: Superficial and deep dissection using medial parapatellar approach.

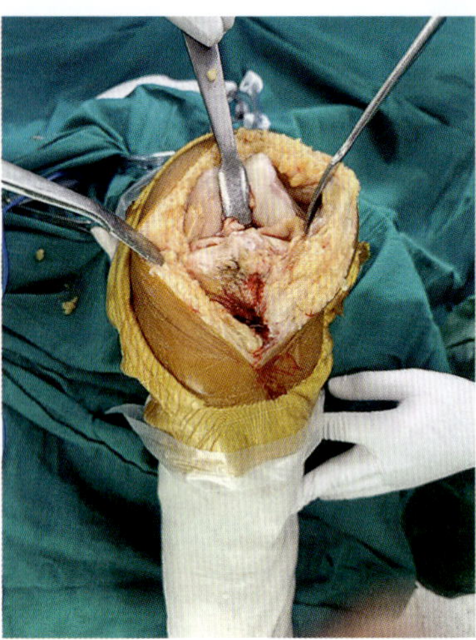

FIG. 3: Placement of bony spikes: Medial, lateral, and posterior to tibial surface.

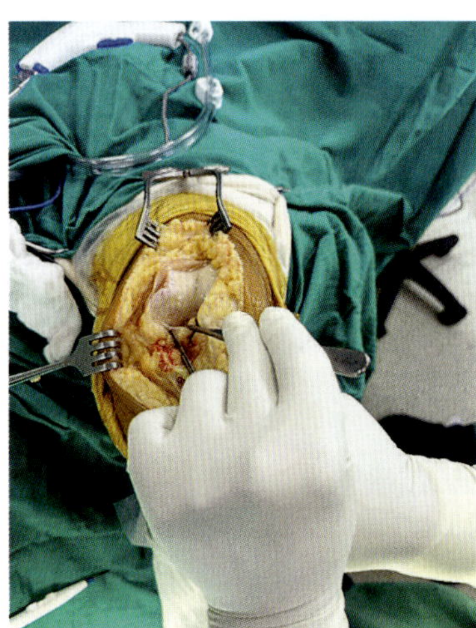

FIG. 4: Excision of menisci and fat pad.

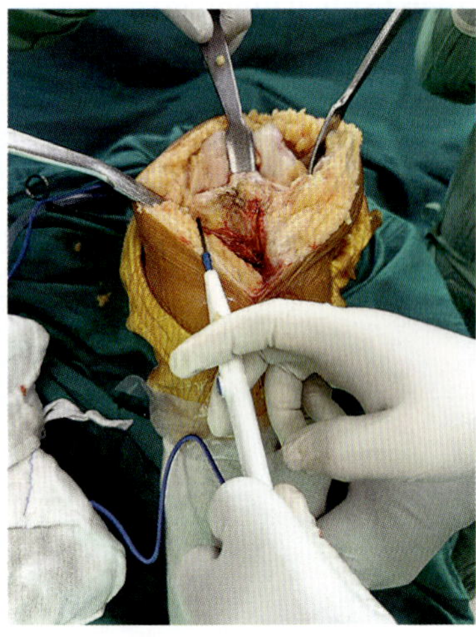

FIG. 5: Posteromedial release (depicted by complete exposure of posteromedial tibial corner).

(PCL)], *where PCL sacrificing designs are used* retropatellar fat pad obstructing surgical view, osteophytes, and inflamed synovial tissue **(Fig. 4)**.

Soft tissue release: Posteromedial tibial soft tissue release is essential **(Fig. 5)** *[except in severe valgus knees with lax medial* *collateral ligaments (MCLs)],* and lateral patellofemoral ligament is incised.

PATELLAR EVERSION/SUBLUXATION

Proximal Tibial Bone Cut

- Extramedullary jig is placed aligning the medial one-third of the tibial tuberosity to the center of the ankle joint (this line also passes along the tibial shin and through the axis of the second metatarsal, with the ankle in neutral position) **(Fig. 6)**.
- Alignment rod confirms mechanical axis placement of this jig.
- Stylus is affixed to jig with two pins (at 0 mark), aimed to cut either 9 mm (from normal unaffected lateral tibial plateau), or 2 mm (from the affected medial tibial plateau); using slotted or nonslotted guides **(Fig. 7)** (*these steps are no longer needed in computer- and robotic-assisted surgery*).
- The first tibial cut is taken with saw and completed with an osteotome; surface is smoothened **(Figs. 8 and 9)**.
- Tibial sizing is now achieved with tibial sizing tray **(Fig. 10)**.

Distal Femoral Bone Cut

- The femoral canal is entered with drill (5 mm anterior to insertion of anterior cruciate ligament on the femoral intercondylar area)

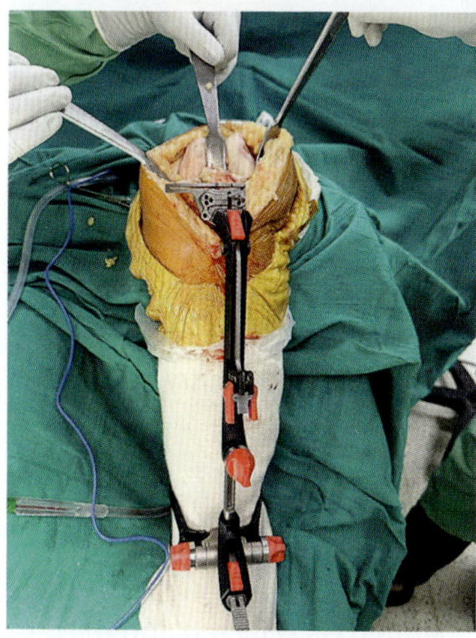

FIG. 6: Placement of extramedullary tibial alignment jig.

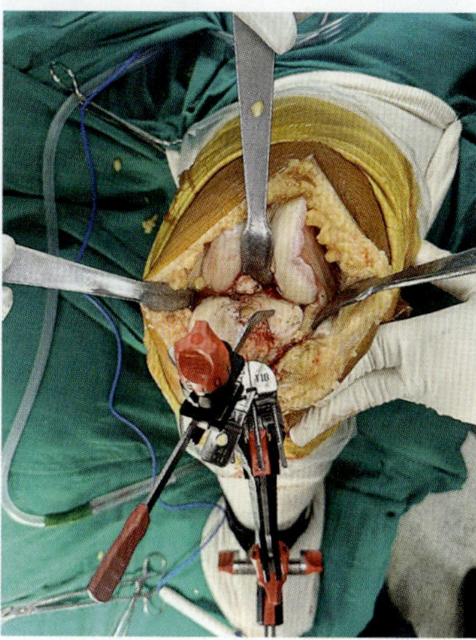

FIG. 7: Confirmation of level of tibial cut with stylus.

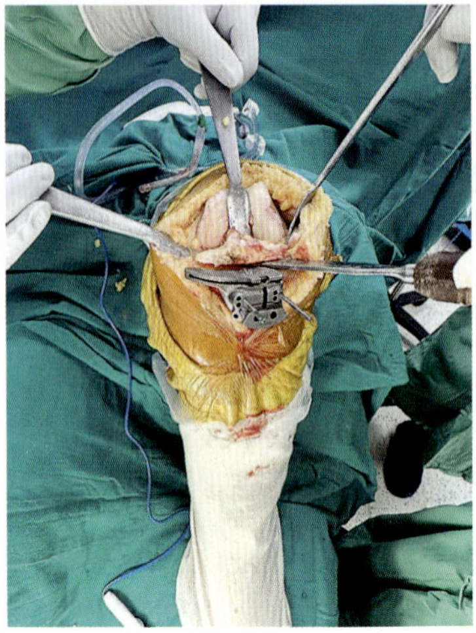

FIG. 8: Proximal tibial cut taken with saw and eased out with osteotome.

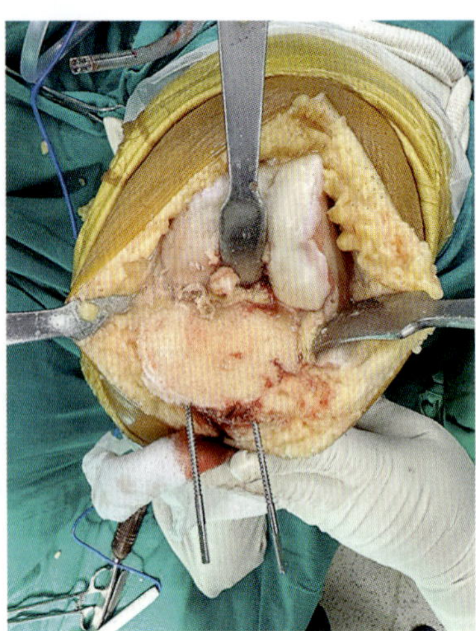

FIG. 9: Proximal tibial cut achieved.

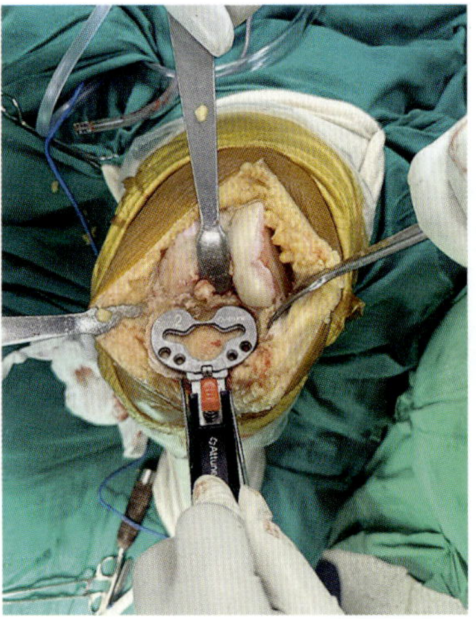

FIG. 10: Tibial sizing with trial tibial tray.

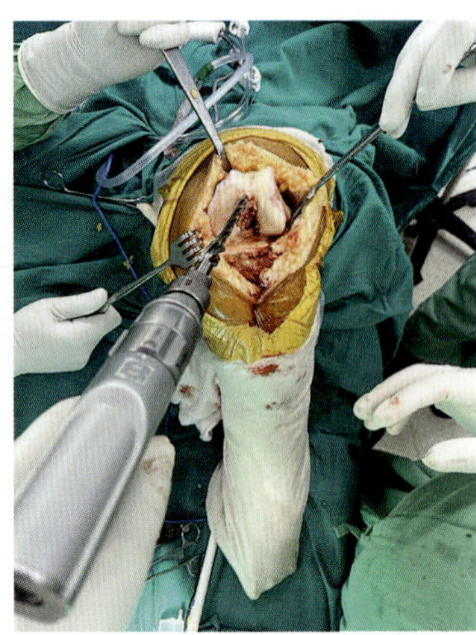

FIG. 11: Femoral entry with drill.

and widened. The canal is washed to remove bony debris and loose marrow fat **(Fig. 11)**.

- Intramedullary jig is inserted into femoral canal with 5–7° valgus angulation, and 9-mm distal cut (slotted) is selected and fixed to the anterior surface of the distal femur with pins **(Figs. 12 and 13)**.

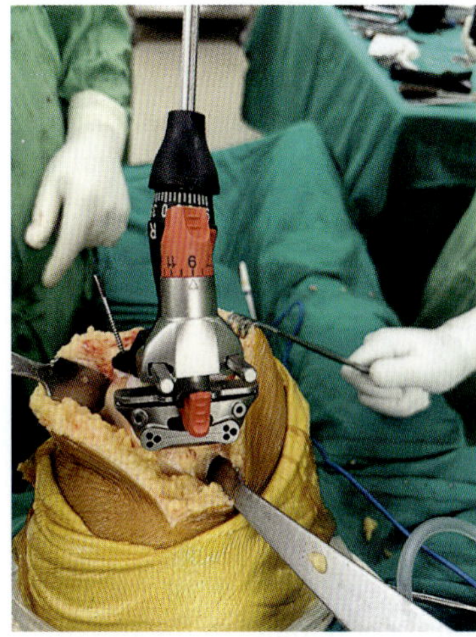

FIG. 12: Intramedullary femoral jig aligning distal femoral cutting block at 5–7° valgus angle.

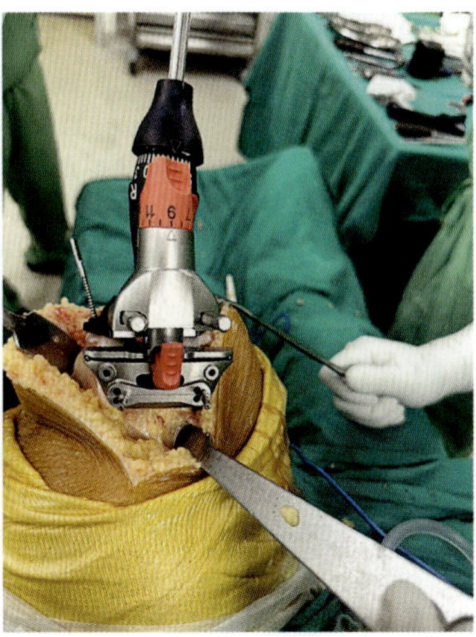

FIG. 13: Distal femur cutting block set to desired level of cut and fixed with pins.

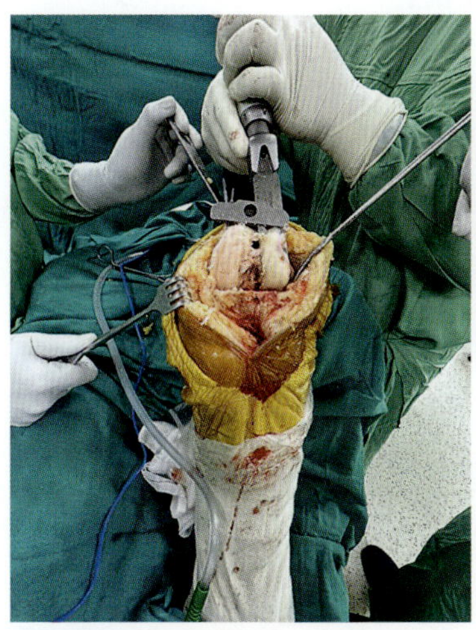

FIG. 14: Intramedullary jig removed and distal femoral cut taken.

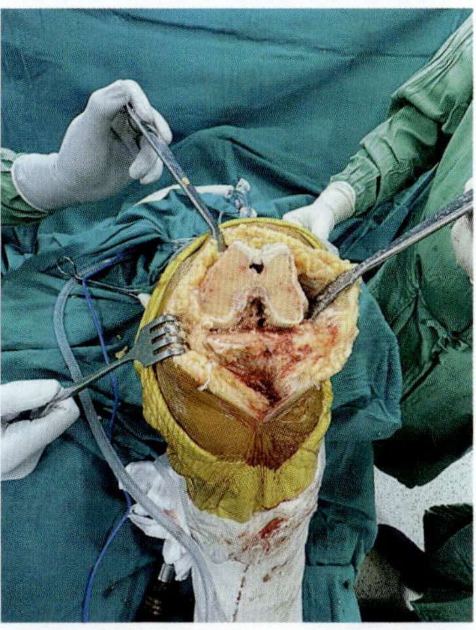

FIG. 15: Distal femoral cut achieved.

- Alignment can be confirmed with an alignment rod inserted onto the jig.
- Intramedullary rod with distal valgus jig is extracted.
- Distal femoral cut is completed **(Figs. 14 and 15)**.

Femoral Component Sizing (and Rotation)

- The femoral sizing jig is placed on flat cut distal surface of femur and the femoral component sized, at the same time the insertion points of the AP cutting jig are marked. Medial pin slot is anterior and lateral pin slot is posterior, and thus, the line joining these points is angulated 3° to the posterior intercondylar line (horizontal), providing the 3° external rotation needed for ensuring a rectangular flexion gap.
- Femoral component rotation is *confirmed* by using either the transepicondylar axis (ensuring that the posterior femoral cut is parallel to a line drawn between the medial and lateral femoral epicondyles), anteroposterior axis (posterior femoral cut perpendicular to this axis), posterior femoral condyles (3° of external rotation off a line between them), or the cut surface of the proximal tibia (posterior femoral cut parallel to the proximal tibial cut in flexion, after the soft tissues have been balanced in extension) **(Fig. 16)**.

Anteroposterior Femoral Bone Cuts

- Appropriate size AP cutting jig is then placed into the pin marks created on the distal surface and fixed **(Fig. 17)**. Alternatively, Ranawat's jig may be used (to make the anterior-posterior cuts) **(Fig. 18)**.

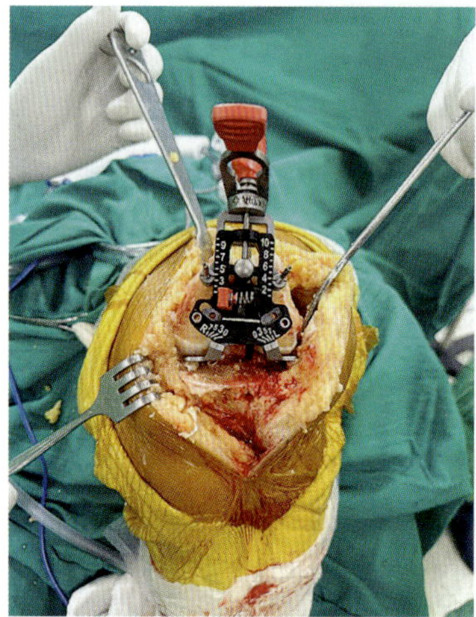

FIG. 16: Femoral sizing jig imparting 3° external rotation to femoral cuts.

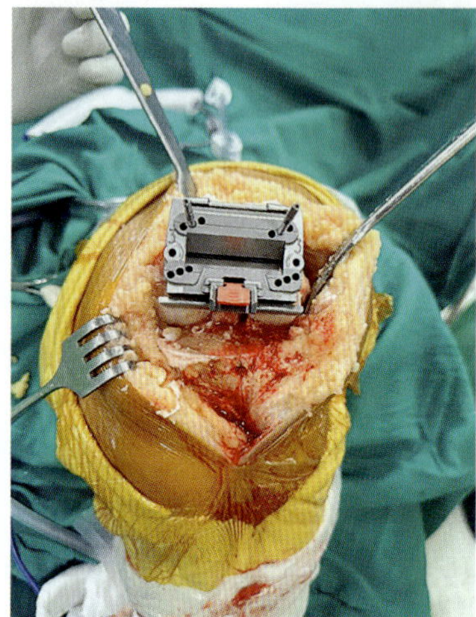

FIG. 17: Placement of AP cutting jig into the pin sites marked by the sizing jig.

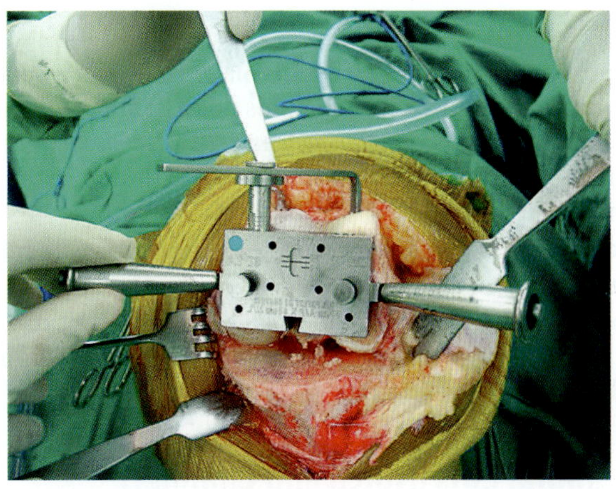

FIG. 18: Ranawat's jig (alternative method) used for sizing.

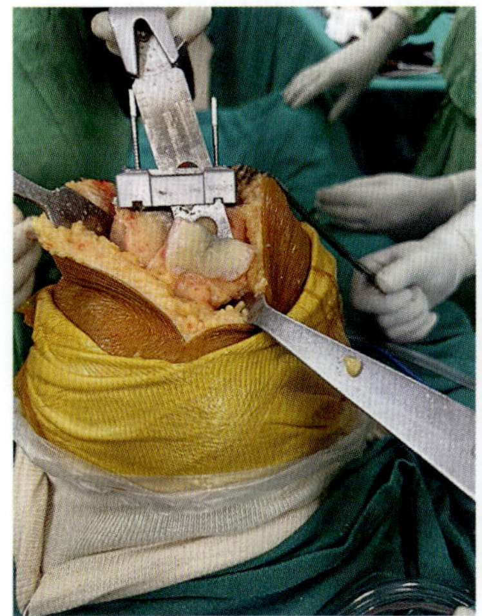

FIG. 19: Anterior femoral cut achieved.

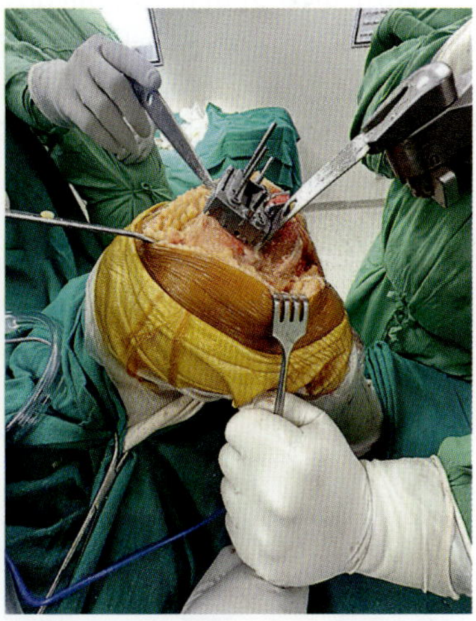

FIG. 20: Posterior femoral cuts achieved.

- Amount to be resected is checked with the angel's wing guide to prevent notching.
- Anterior and posterior cuts are taken (cutting through slots to prevent skiving of the saw blade) **(Figs. 19 and 20)**.

Gap Assessment and Alignment

- An appropriate size spacer block is placed between resected bone ends in flexion and extension at this point in time and checked to be equal and balanced **(Figs. 21 and 22)**. Necessary corrections are made to correct nonrectangularity and flexion/extension gap mismatch, if needed.
- Joint stability in varus-valgus is checked, appropriate releases as required may be carried out **(Fig. 23)**.
- In extension, the femoral and tibial alignment rods are inserted into the spacer block and appropriate mechanical axis achieved (and marked on the tibia).

Final Femoral Cuts (Notch and Chamfer)

- Combined chamfer and notch cutting jig are then placed onto distal femur (ensuring that it sits flat on anterior and distal surfaces and matches the posterior femoral cut) **(Fig. 24)**.
- Notch is prepared using a reciprocating saw blade and completed with osteotomes and hammer **(Figs. 25 and 26)**.
- Chamfers are then cut **(Fig. 27)**.
- Jig is removed and any irregularities shaved and freshened with rasp, if necessary.

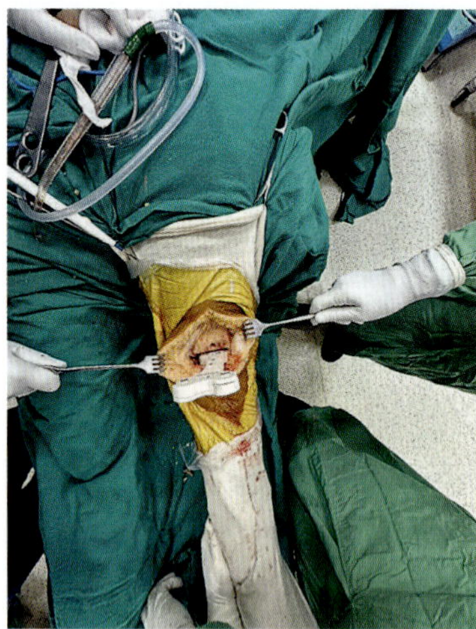

FIG. 21: Checking flexion-extension gap in extension.

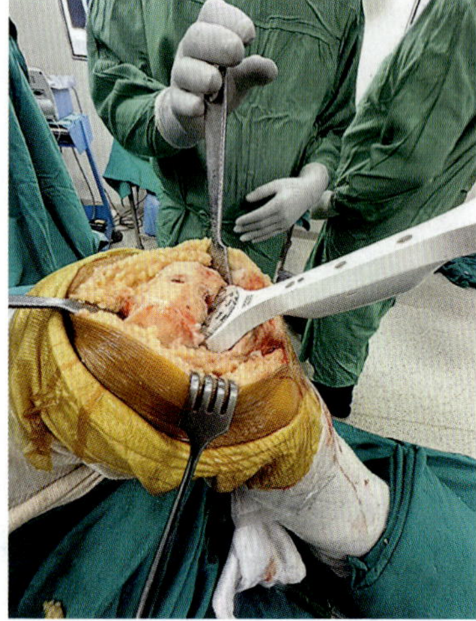

FIG. 22: Checking flexion-extension gap in flexion.

- Remove any medial or lateral osteophytes that tent the collateral ligaments. Remove posterior condylar osteophytes with a curved osteotome (because they can tent the posterior capsule and narrow the extension gap or impinge during knee flexion) **(Fig. 28)**.

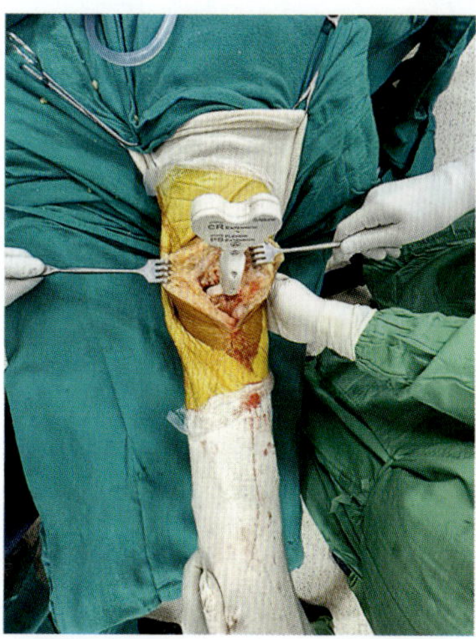

FIG. 23: Checking for varus-valgus stability in extension with spacer block.

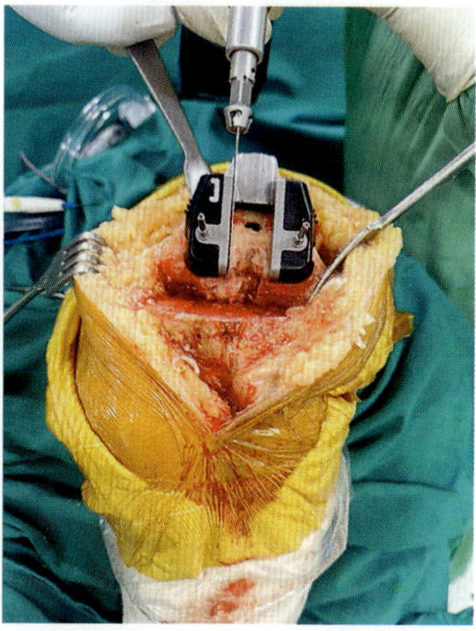

FIG. 24: Placement of combined chamfer-notch cutting jig on distal femur.

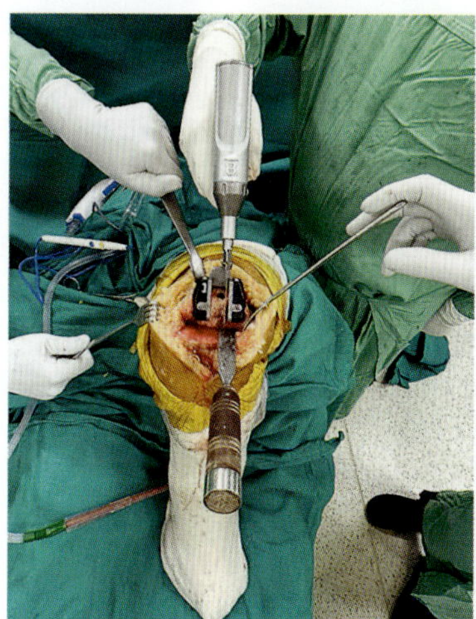

FIG. 25: Cutting of notch with reciprocating saw (in cruciate-substituting designs).

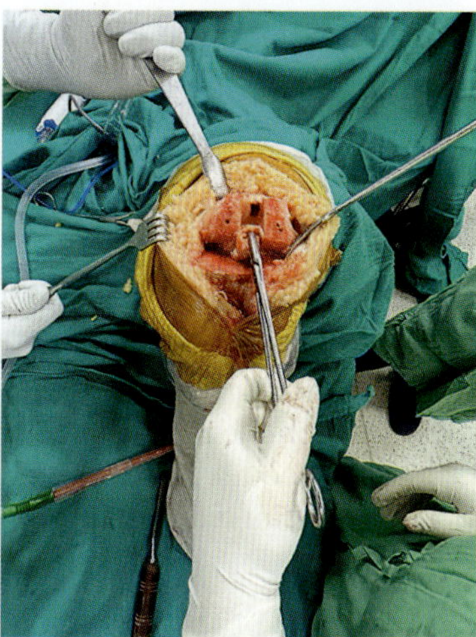

FIG. 26: Excision of femoral intercondylar notch.

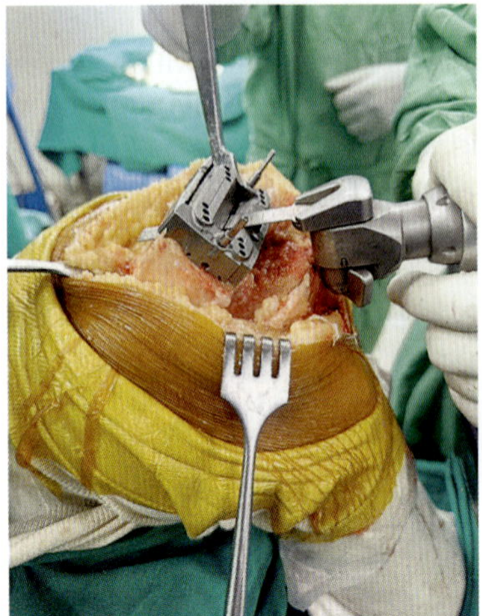

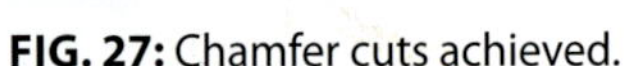

FIG. 27: Chamfer cuts achieved.

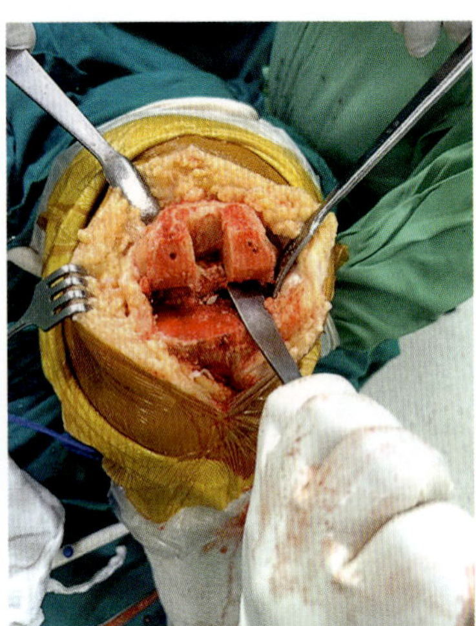

FIG. 28: Removal of posterior osteophytes with osteotome and hammer.

Blocking the Femoral Canal

Bone derived from chamfer cuts is cut, shaped, and punched over the femoral entry point to block the canal (and reduce bone bleed from the marrow) **(Fig. 29)**.

Trial Implantation and Reduction

- Trial femoral implant (prepared size and side) is placed onto the distal cut surface of the femur and gently impacted maintaining flexion at knee joint **(Fig. 30)**.
- If there is incongruent fit, check for oblique/skived cuts, hard sclerotic bone on any surface, impinging posterior osteophytes, or intercondylar notch irregularities, and correct the same.
- Trial tibial tray is similarly placed on tibial surface. Trial tibial insert corresponding on size to tibial tray and 8 mm thickness (with aforementioned described cuts for femur and tibia, 8 mm insert is required to recreate stability) is placed over the tibial tray and the joint reduced **(Fig. 31)**.

Alignment, Stability, and Mobility Check

- Once the knee is straightened, alignment rods are placed in the jig holding the tibial tray and overall mechanical alignment checked in AP and profile views **(Figs. 32 and 33)**.

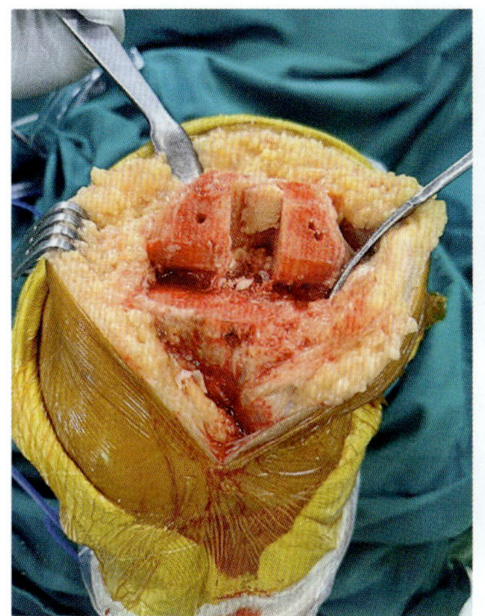

FIG. 29: Removal of jigs and placement of bony block for femoral canal.

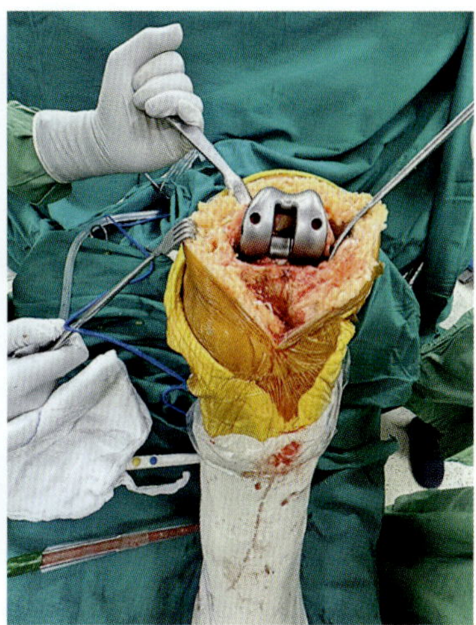

FIG. 30: View of joint with trial femoral implant.

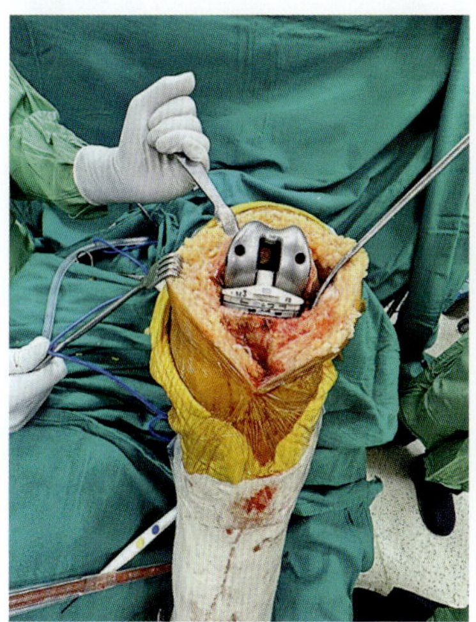

FIG. 31: Placement of trial tibial tray with trial insert.

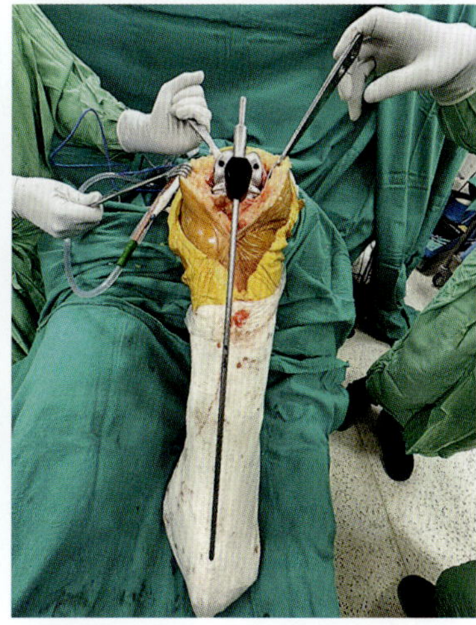

FIG. 32: Alignment rod placed through trial tibial tray—anterior view.

- Varus-valgus balance, anteroposterior stability, and range of movement (ROM) are then checked **(Figs. 34 and 35)**. This can be fine-tuned with medial or lateral soft tissue releases, if needed.

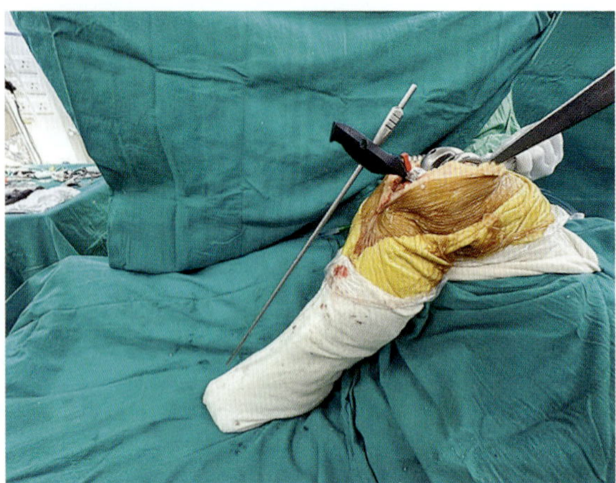

FIG. 33: Alignment rod placed through trial tibial tray—profile view.

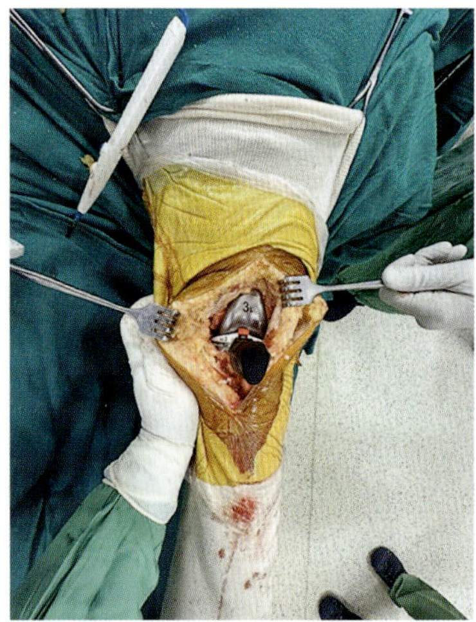

FIG. 34: Checking stability with trial implants—varus stress.

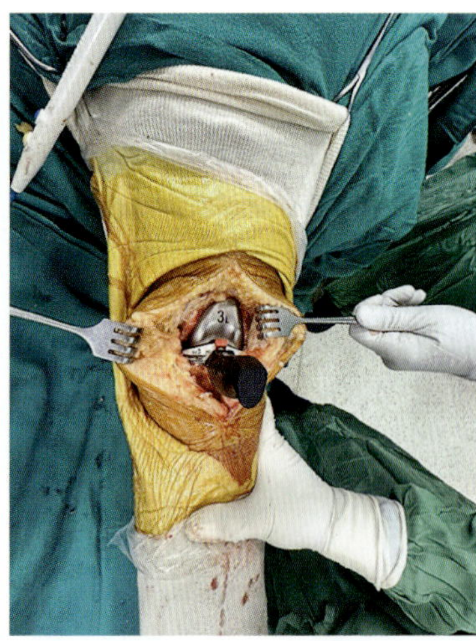

FIG. 35: Checking stability with trial implants—valgus stress.

- The knee stability and alignment are then checked in flexion, and appropriate tibial rotational alignment is attained and marked with cautery (the tibial tray holding jig may need to be externally rotated to achieve this) **(Fig. 36)**.
- After bone deficiencies have been treated, ligamentous balancing is satisfactory, and the extensor mechanism is tracking properly, the trial components are removed.

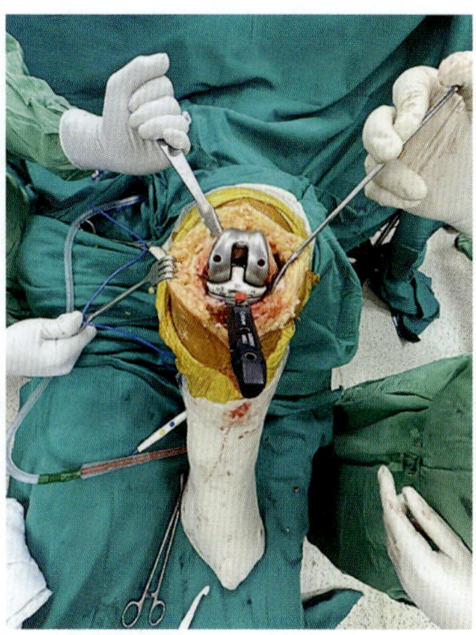

FIG. 36: Rotational alignment of tibial tray finalized and marked with cautery.

Final Tibial Preparation

- Knee is flexed, the tibia gently displaced anteriorly (with appropriately placed posterior, medial, and lateral Hohmann's retractors).
- Selected size tibial tray jig is placed on surface to cover the maximum tibial surface area and aligned to marked cautery point **(Fig. 37)**.
- Central hole is drilled in tibial canal and is made for the peg as per the jig **(Fig. 38)**.
- This jig is then removed. Keel punch is inserted into jig to attain keel cuts **(Fig. 39)**.
- Tibial tray jig (along with keel jig) is then removed and all prepared surfaces washed and dried **(Fig. 40)**.
- With sclerotic bone surfaces, a 2.5/3.2 mm drill bit can be used to make multiple perforations into the underlying cancellous bone (femur or tibia) to allow cement intrusion.

Patella Preparation (Replacement/Patellaplasty) and Patellofemoral Tracking Check

Replacement

- Patella is everted, its circumference lightly cauterized, and osteophytes excised **(Figs. 41 and 42)**.

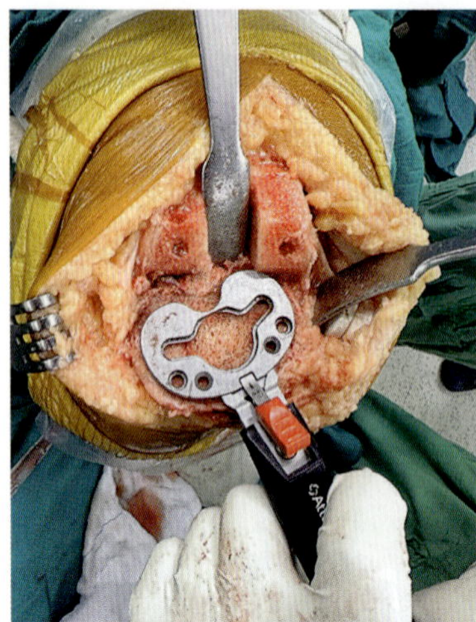

FIG. 37: Placement of tibial preparation jig on surface (as marked with cautery).

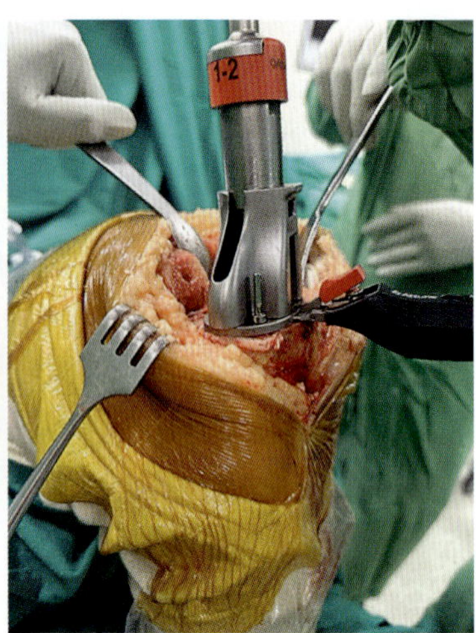

FIG. 38: Drill hole being made in tibia through jig.

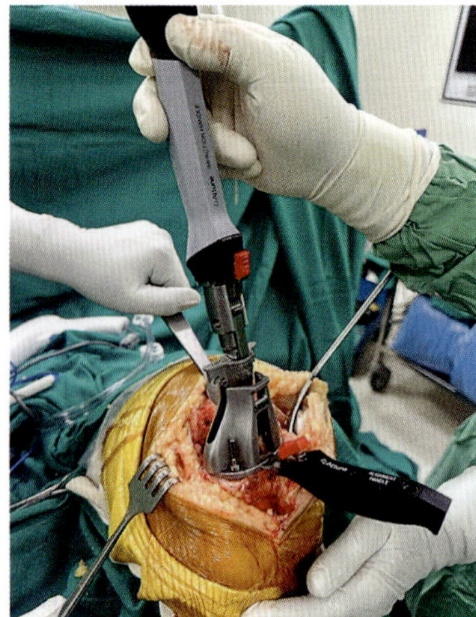

FIG. 39: Keel punch being driven into tibial surface through jig.

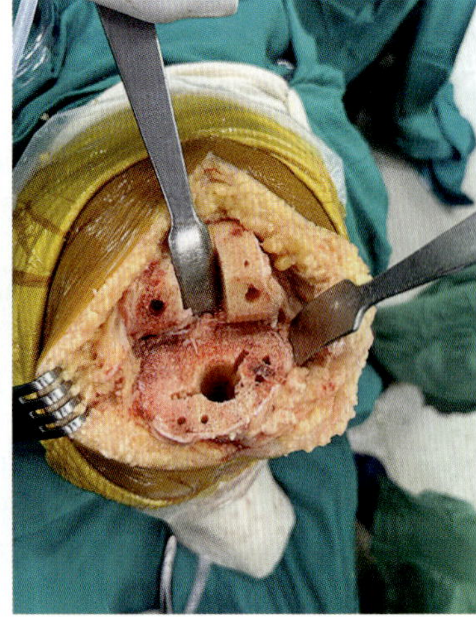

FIG. 40: Prepared femoral and tibial surfaces.

- Patella thickness is measured using vernier calipers **(Fig. 43)**.
- Patellar jaw clamp is then applied to hold patella, and patellar surface is shaved off leaving 13–15 mm of patellar bone intact **(Figs. 44 and 45)**.

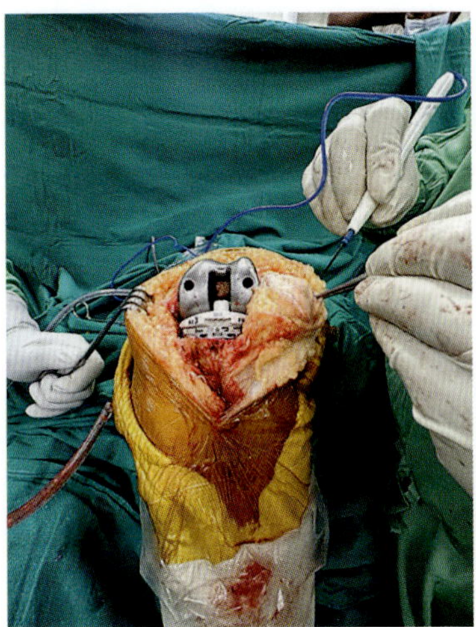

FIG. 41: Light cauterization of peripatellar synovium.

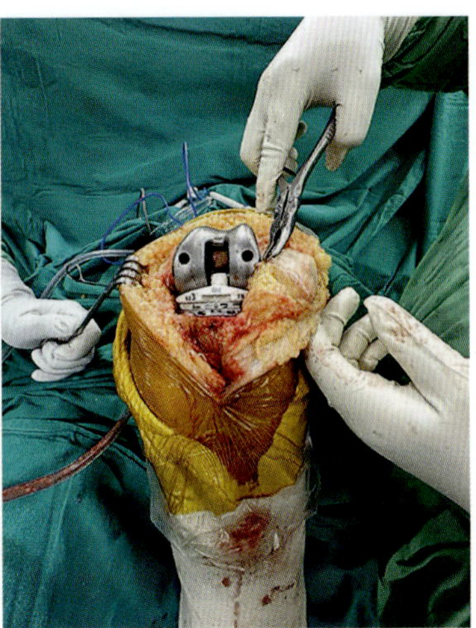

FIG. 42: Excision of patellar osteophytes.

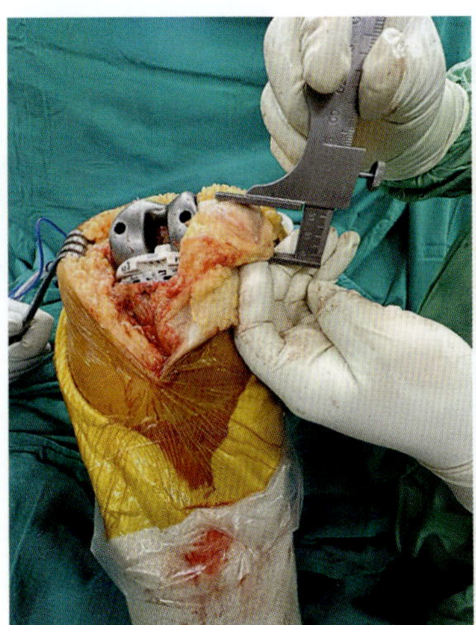

FIG. 43: Measurement of patellar thickness using vernier calipers.

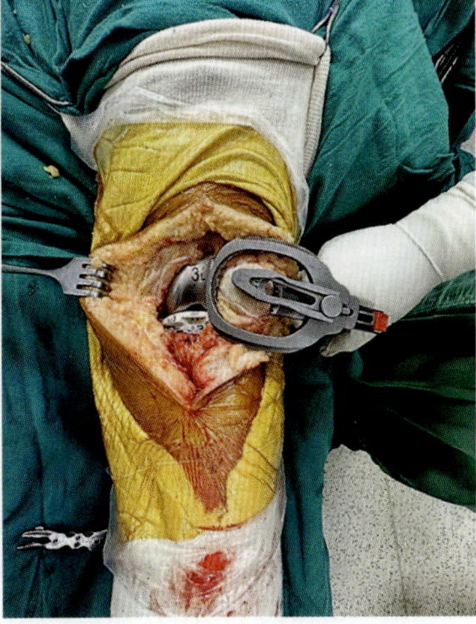

FIG. 44: Patellar jaw clamp holding patella at desired level for cut.

- Patellar jig is then placed on surface, and drill holes (two placed medially and one on lateral part of the patella) are made to accept patellar prosthesis, with the aim of mildly translating the jig plate medially for better patellar tracking **(Fig. 46)**.

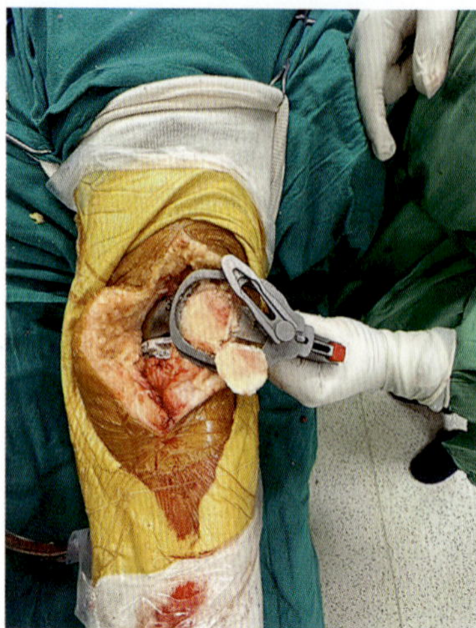

FIG. 45: Patellar surface being cut at desired level for patellar button implantation.

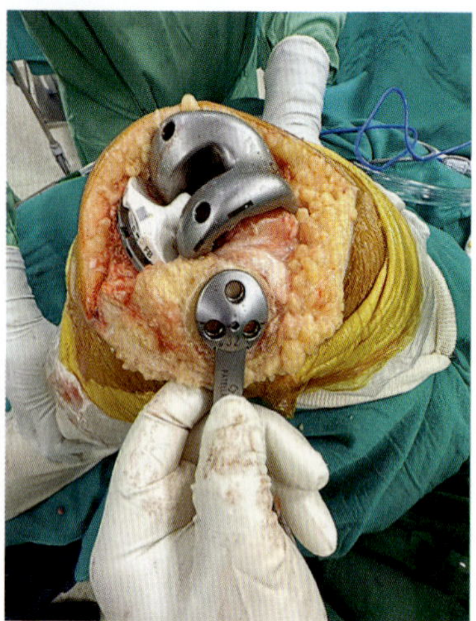

FIG. 46: Preparation of patellar surface to accept pegs of patellar button.

- Trial patellar button is placed onto the prepared surface and patellofemoral tracking checked **(Figs. 47 and 48)**.

Patellaplasty

Patellar surface is gently shaved to remove worn out cartilage. Leave smooth subchondral bony surfaces which are gently sloped on the medial and lateral surfaces (without irregularities) **(Figs. 49 and 50)**.

Wound Lavage

- The entire bony surface is lavaged using pulsatile lavage system to expose the porous surfaces (thus enhancing bone-cement interlock) and remove blood clots and fat droplets **(Fig. 51)**.
- The surface is then dried and covered with sponges to accept cement **(Fig. 52)**.

Final Component Implantation

- Usually, tibial implantation is done before implanting the femur in posterior-stabilized (PS) designs. However, patellar cementation can be done (even before the tibia) and the implant held onto the patella with the patellar clamp **(Figs. 53 and 54)**.

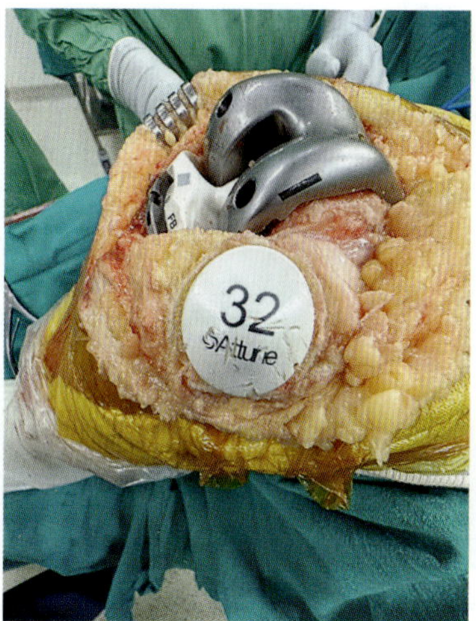

FIG. 47: Placement of trial patellar button.

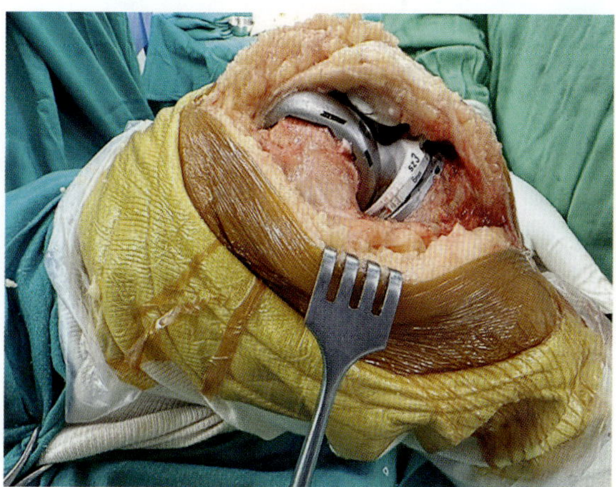

FIG. 48: Patellofemoral tracking checked with trial implants.

- The tibial component (undersurface) is coated with the prepared cement, held with the impactor, and hammered into the prepared tibial surface. Excess cement is cleared off from the periphery of the implant **(Figs. 55 to 57)**.
- Cement is then applied in a layer along the prepared femoral surfaces (including notch), and the femoral component (where closed box systems are used) is impacted maintaining

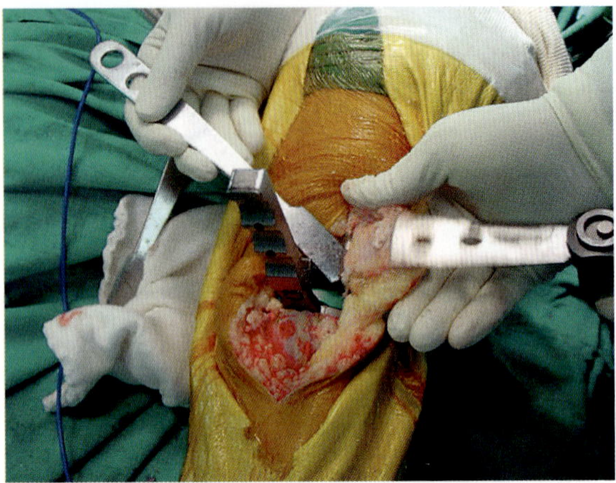

FIG. 49: Patellar surface being shaved (patellaplasty).

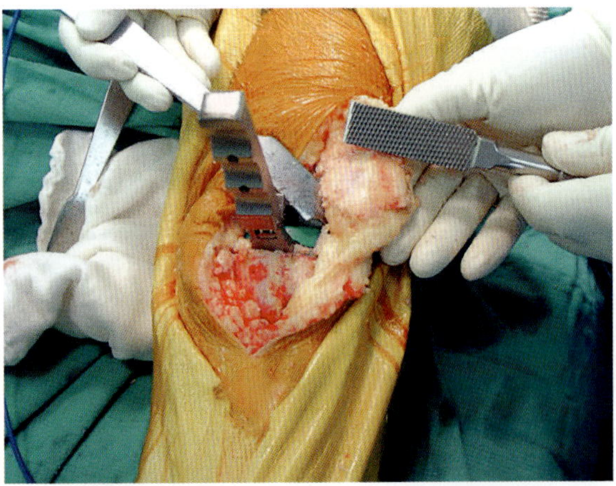

FIG. 50: Smooth patellar surface postpatellaplasty.

component extension. To minimize the amount of cement to be removed from the posterior femoral recesses, cement can be applied to the posterior condylar fixation surfaces of the femoral prosthesis rather than to the bone. Excess cement is cleared off from the implant margins **(Figs. 58 to 60)**.

Trial insert is placed onto the tibial tray and the joint reduced and checked flexion and extension **(Figs. 61 and 62)**.

- The trial tibial insert that gives adequate varus and valgus stability in full extension should be used. If a *thinner trial spacer*

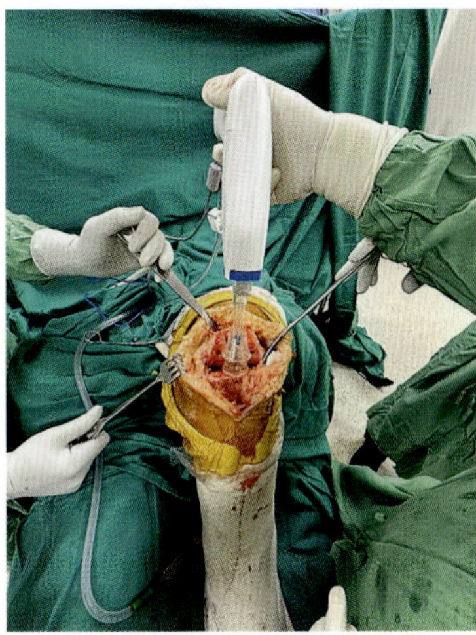

FIG. 51: Pulsatile lavage used to flush out clots and fat from prepared bone surfaces.

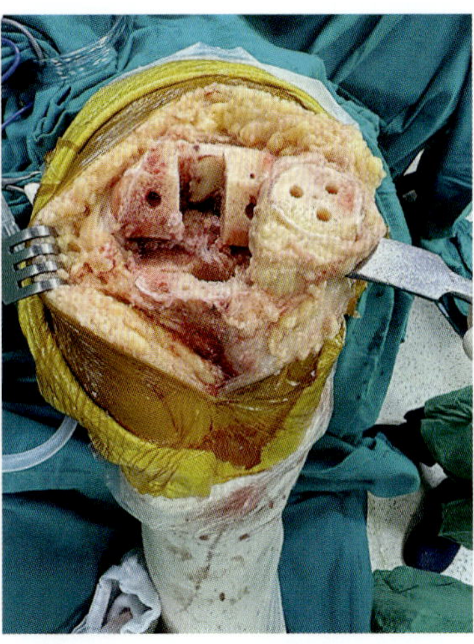

FIG. 52: Surfaces ready to accept bone cement (postpulsatile lavage).

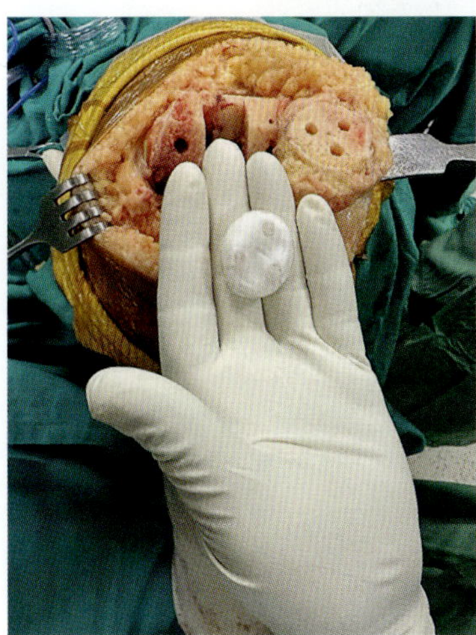

FIG. 53: Bone cement applied to patellar implant undersurface.

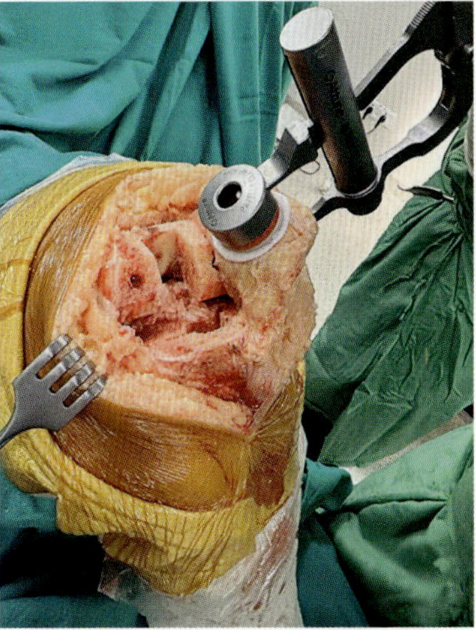

FIG. 54: Patellar implant affixed to prepared patellar surface with patellar clamp.

is substituted, hyperextension of the knee and posterior liftoff of the tibial component could result. Also, extending the knee over a *thicker trial spacer* before final cement polymerization can impact the components into soft bone.

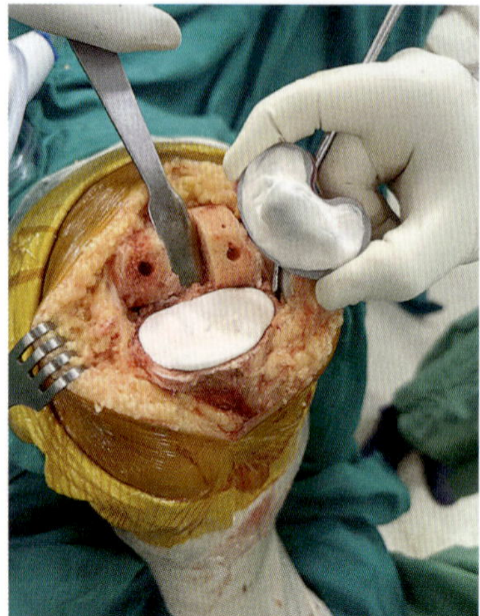

FIG. 55: Preparation of tibial implant and tibial surface with bone cement.

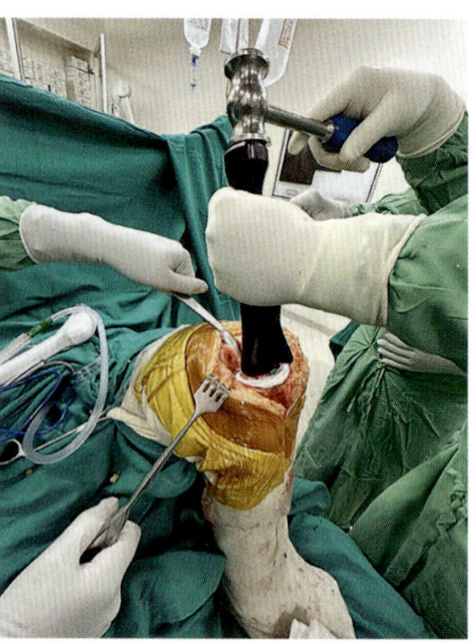

FIG. 56: Impaction of tibial implant onto prepared tibial surface.

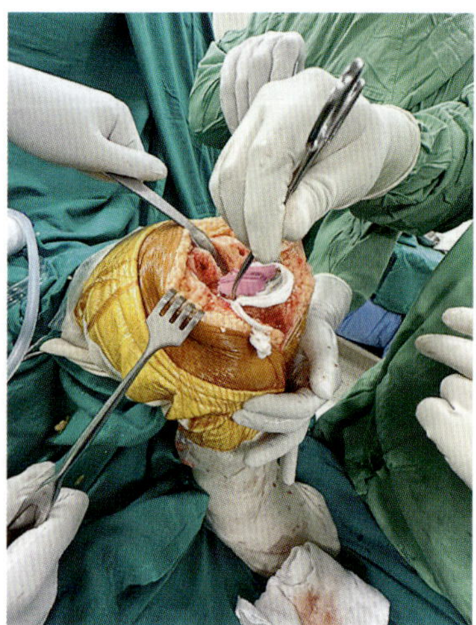

FIG. 57: Removal of excess cement from periphery of tibial implant.

- While the cement sets, the knee is kept in 0° extension (through sustained pressure anteriorly) and excess cement removed **(Fig. 62)**.
- Care must be taken not to hyperextend the knee because the joint is then unstable, and the posterior neurovascular structures can be injured.

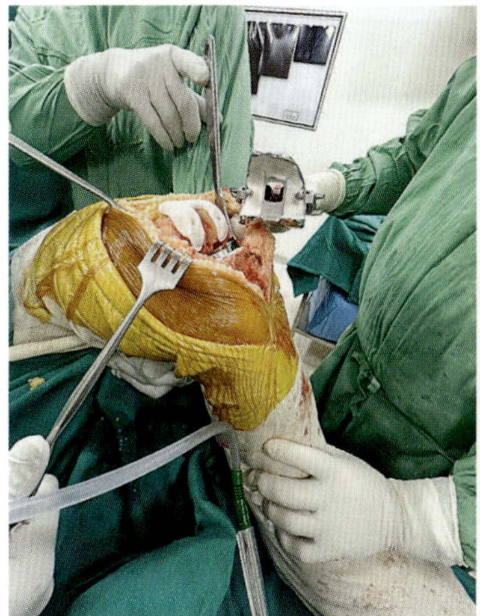

FIG. 58: Preparation of femoral implant and femoral surface with bone cement.

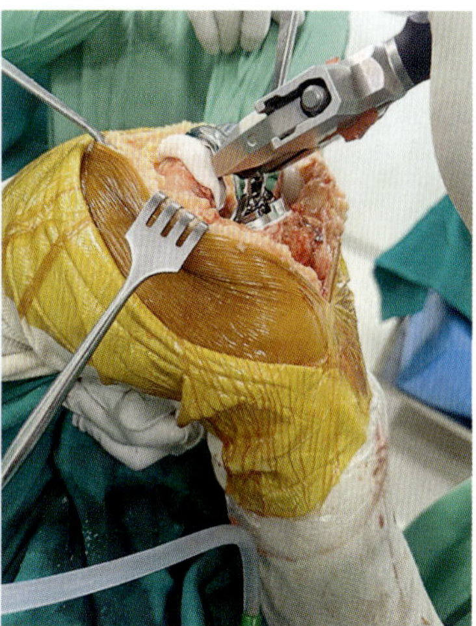

FIG. 59: Impaction of femoral implant onto prepared femoral surface.

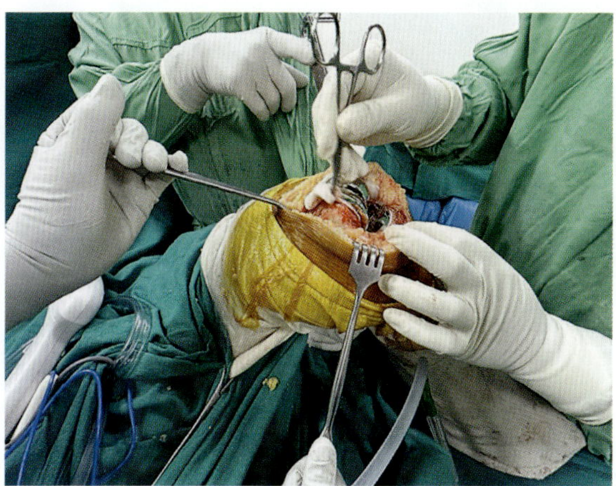

FIG. 60: Removal of excess cement from periphery of femoral implant.

- Once the cement sets, trial insert is removed. A meticulous search for any bone or cement debris should be made before implantation of the final tibial ultra-high molecular weight polyethylene (UHMWPE).
- The actual tibial insert is then eased into the tibial tray using the insertion device **(Figs. 63 and 64)**.

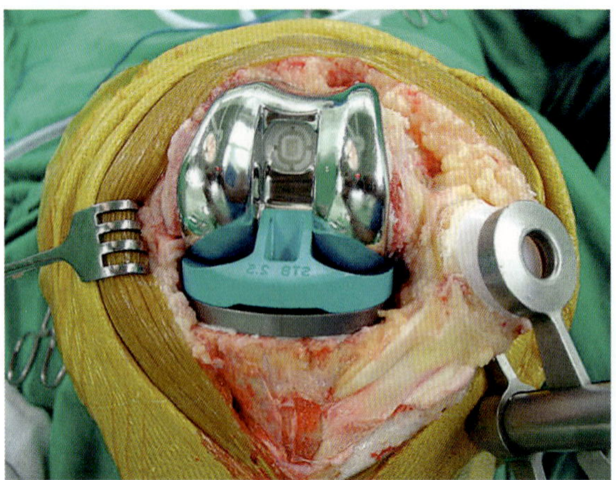

FIG. 61: Trial spacer inserted, and reduction checked in flexion.

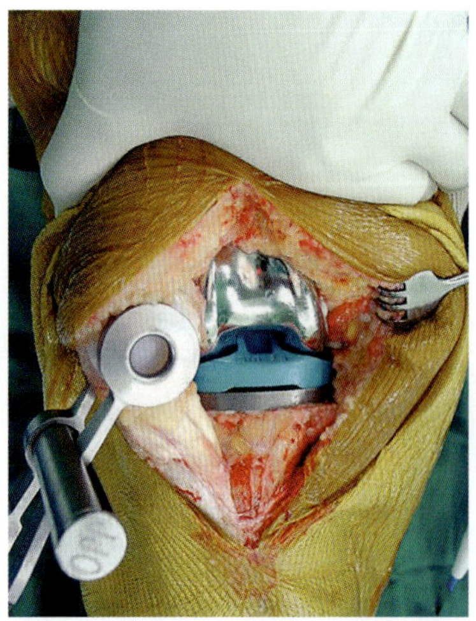

FIG. 62: Position of the implants in extension while the cement is setting.

Joint Reduction and Final Check

- The joint is then reduced and the joint checked once again for stability (anterior-posterior and varus-valgus) and mobility (range of motion and flexion-extension tightness) **(Fig. 65)**.
- Patellar tracking is confirmed using the "no thumb" test **(Fig. 66)**.

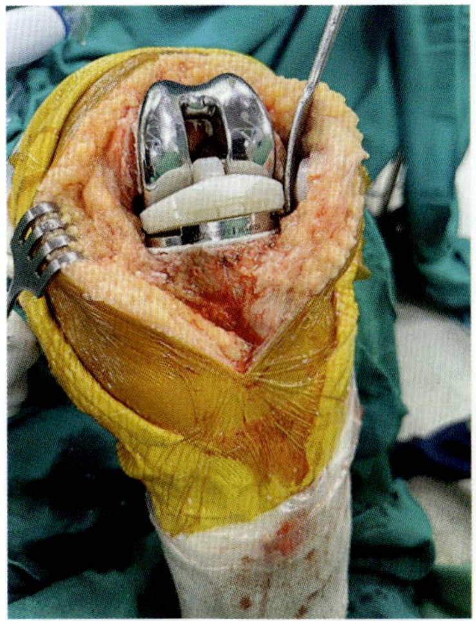

FIG. 63: Final insert placed onto tibial tray.

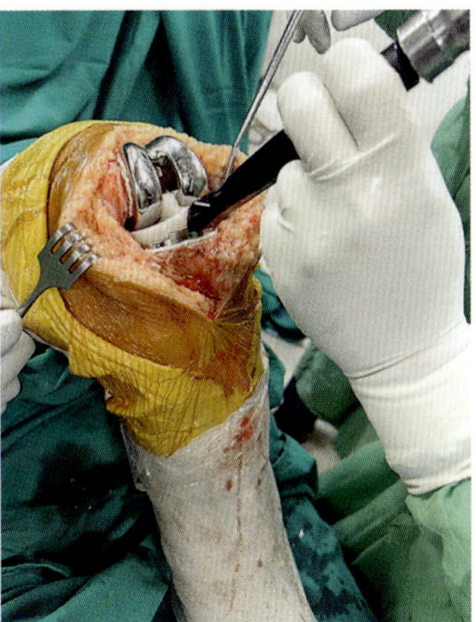

FIG. 64: Final insert seated onto tibial tray with insertion device.

Wound Closure

- The wound is once again lavaged with saline and rechecked for bleeders, which are cauterized.
- Drains may be used, and the wound is sutured in layers using no. 1 and 2-0 vicryl in 30° flexion.
- Retinaculum is sutured with 1 vicryl using interrupted vertical mattress stitches (aligning the cut ends anatomically), and the subcutaneous tissue sutured with 2-0 vicryl using interrupted or continuous interlocking stitches **(Fig. 67)**.
- Skin incision is closed with staples (drain stitch is applied where used).

Dressing

- 25 × 10 mm Curapore/Tegaderm dressing is placed on the wound, and Robert-Jones compression bandage (with two layers of wool and crepe) is then applied from ankle to mid-thigh level **(Figs. 68 and 69)**.
- Tourniquet is usually released at this time and distal pulses checked.
- Some surgeons prefer to deflate the tourniquet, check bleeders, and re-inflate it only for cementing the components.

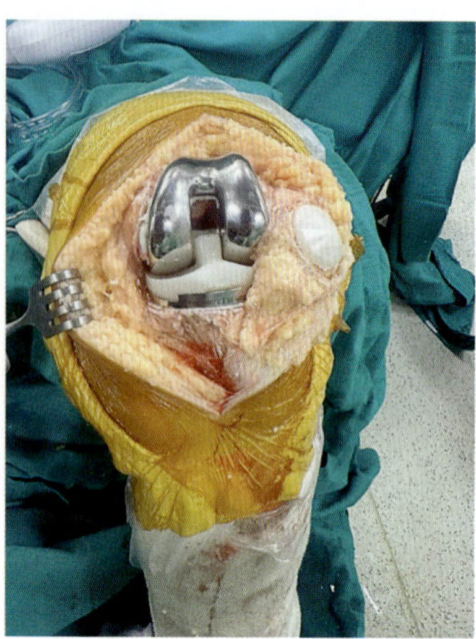

FIG. 65: View of final implant positions with everted patella.

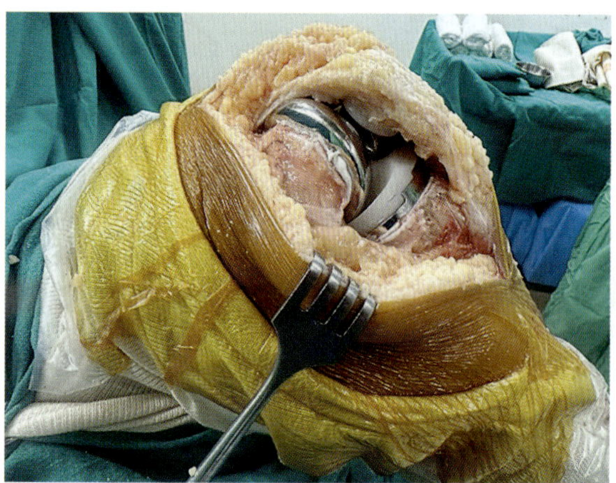

FIG. 66: Patellar tracking checking using "no thumb" test.

For *cementless fixation* of total knee components, the technique of implantation involves preparation of the cut bone surfaces with far more accuracy and precision than with cement fixation. Cementless fixation relies on intimate apposition of the fixation surface to the cut bone surfaces, as well as rigid immediate fixation to minimize micromotion. In experimental models, bone-prosthesis gaps of more than 0.5 mm tend to fill with fibrous tissue (*to offset this, Hofmann*

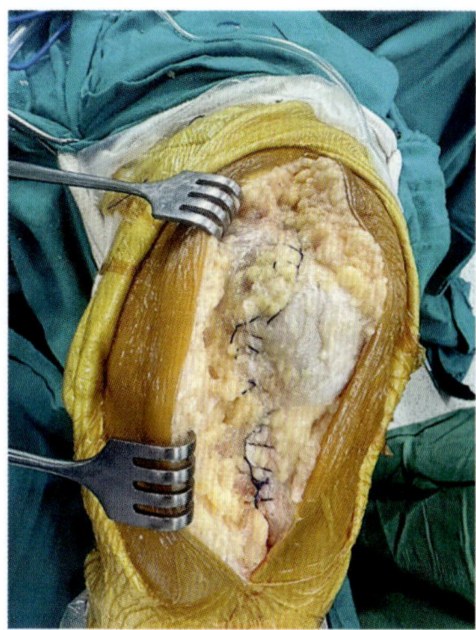

FIG. 67: Medial retinacular closure.

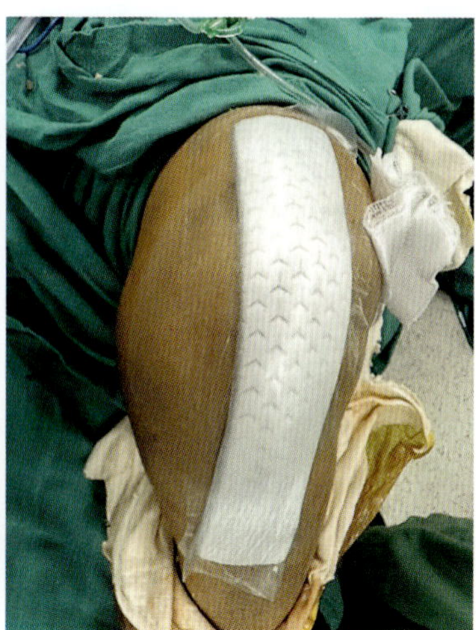

FIG. 68: Curapore/Tegaderm dressing and drain.

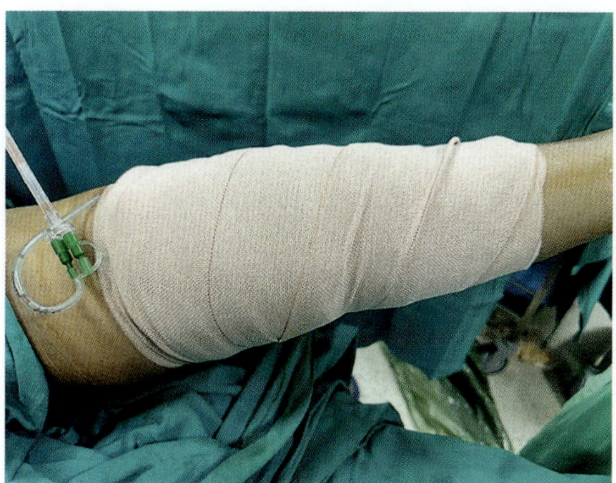

FIG. 69: Robert–Jones compression bandage applied from thigh to ankle.

advocated the use of a fine autogenous bone graft on the upper surface of the tibia to level small irregularities, and Whiteside developed an intramedullary rotary planning tool to obtain a flat upper tibial surface). Retrieval studies have repeatedly demonstrated maximal bone ingrowth around fixation screws and pegs, and the use of such adjunctive fixation is crucial to obtain the stability necessary for bone ingrowth and long-term prosthesis fixation.

Chapter 12

Surgical Technique: Varus Deformity

Varus deformity is the most common deformity of the osteoarthritic knee (**Figs. 1 to 6**).

- *Biomechanics*:
  - Altered anatomical axis: Proximal tibial articular surface is worn medially → increased proximal tibial varus.
  - Altered biomechanical axis: Mechanical axis passing medial to knee joint center.
- Patient position, incision, approach, and exposure similar to standard knee. The initial exposure should include release of the deep portion of the medial collateral ligament (MCL) off the tibia

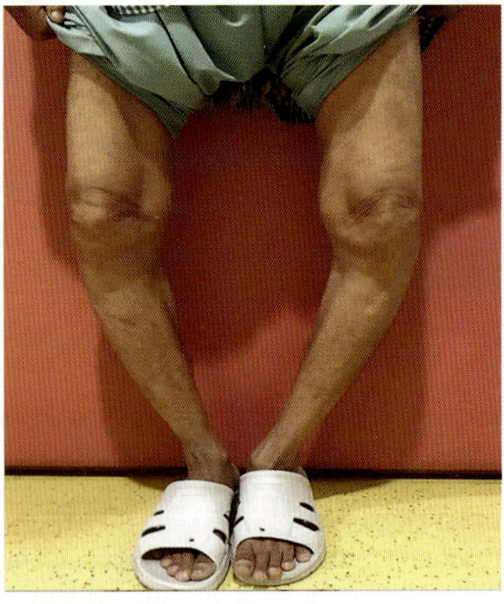

FIG. 1: Clinical photograph of patient with varus knee deformity.

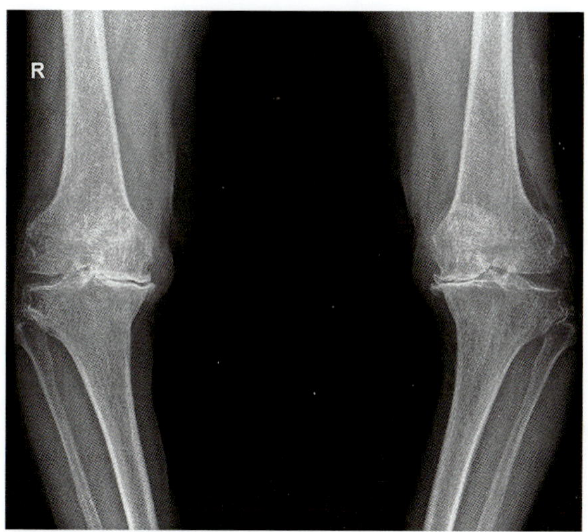

FIG. 2: X-rays of a typical patient with varus knee deformities.

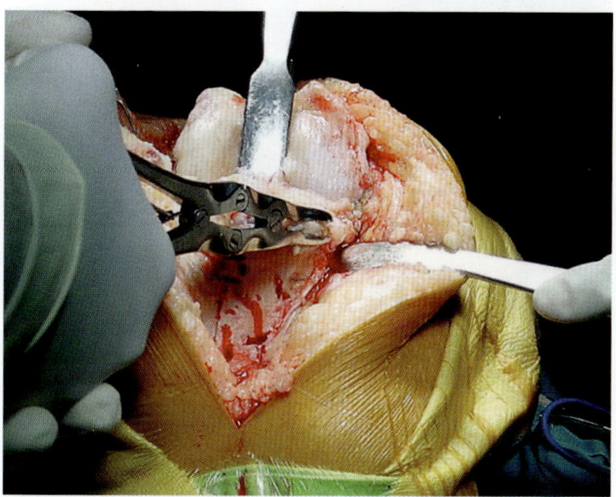

FIG. 3: Excision of protruding medial tibial and femoral osteophytes.

all the way to the posteromedial corner. Osteophytes on both the femur and tibia must be removed completely (they can tent the medial soft tissue sleeve and effectively shorten the MCL).

- *Bone cuts*: The bone cuts follow the same principles as for standard knee, with care being taken to remove 9 mm of bone from the tibial surface (referencing the less affected lateral tibial surface).

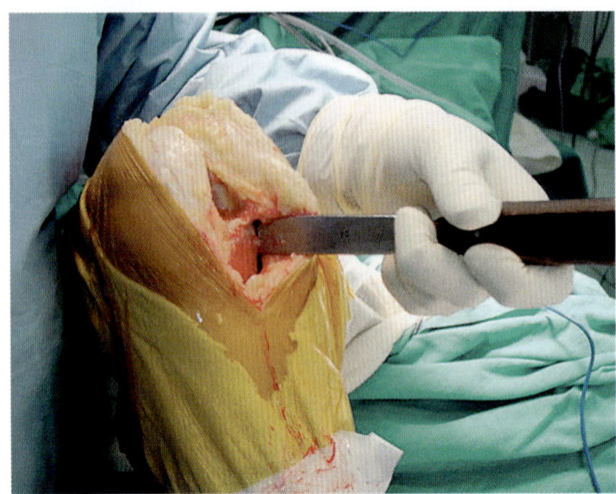

FIG. 4: Posteromedial release [including erasing medial collateral ligament (MCL) insertion] with osteotome.

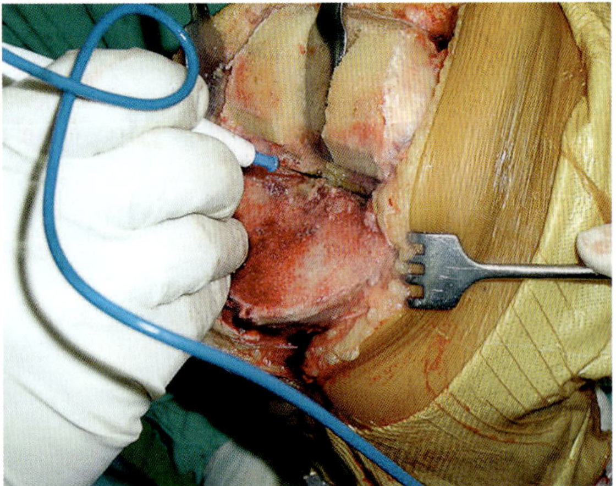

FIG. 5: Posteromedial corner release (with cautery) in severe varus deformity.

Defects, if any, left on the medial tibial plateau can be filled up and managed.

- *Soft tissue balancing*:
  - If a medial contracture persists, the semimembranosus aponeurosis, superficial MCL, and pes anserinus insertions are sequentially released, checking for stability between each stage.

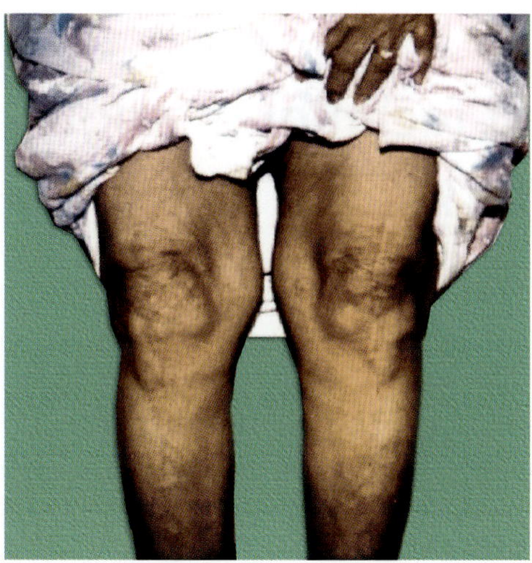

FIG. 6: Postoperative clinical photograph of patient with preoperative varus deformity.

- If the posterior cruciate ligament (PCL) has been preserved and the medial contracture has not been corrected, it can be released at this stage along with the posteromedial capsule, and conversion to a PCL-substituting prosthesis is indicated.
- For persistent, severe medial contracture, with or without lateral attenuation, the periosteum of the tibia can be stripped distally for an additional 4–5 cm, fractionally severing the periosteum at this level if necessary. *This last release rarely is necessary, and care should be taken to avoid overzealous release as that can cause subsequent valgus instability.*

- *Patellofemoral tracking*: Patellar tracking is rarely affected by varus deformity and therefore usually follows the same pattern as that of a normal knee.
- Wound closure
- Closure of the surgical wound in the same fashion as that for the standard knee

Chapter 13

Surgical Technique: Valgus Deformity

Valgus deformity occurs in rheumatoid arthritis and in osteoarthritis with hypoplasia of the lateral femoral condyle **(Figs. 1 and 2)**.

- *Biomechanics*:
    - Altered anatomical axis: Proximal tibial/distal femoral articular surface is worn laterally; proximal tibial valgus/distal femoral increased valgus.
    - Altered biomechanical axis: Mechanical axis passing lateral to knee joint center **(Fig. 3)**.
- *Patient position, incision, approach, and exposure*: Position, incision, and approach are ideally the same even in valgus knees, unless the valgus deformity is very severe (*in which case, a lateral*

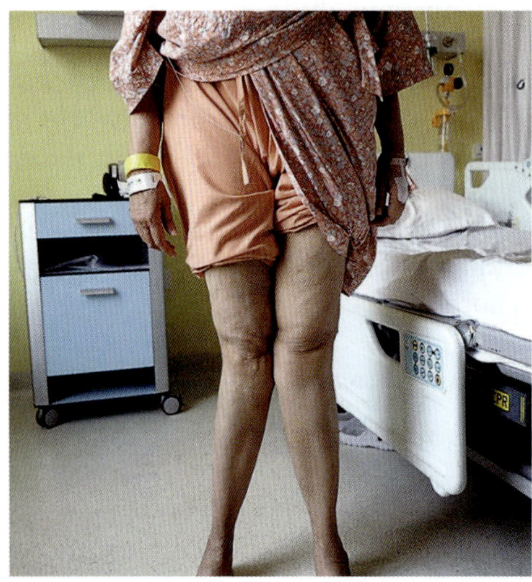

FIG. 1: Clinical photograph of patient with valgus knee deformities.

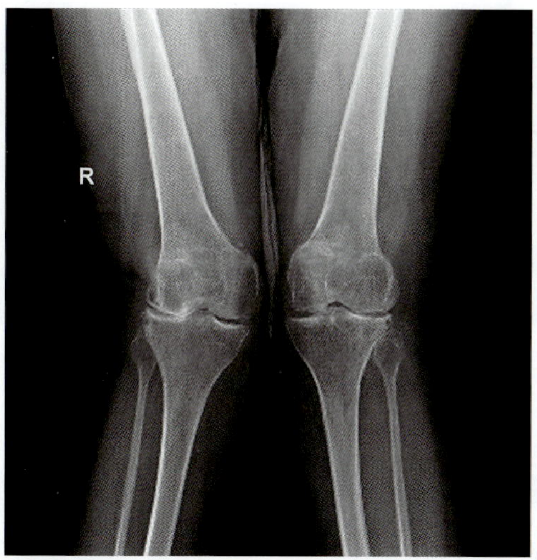

FIG. 2: X-rays of a typical patient with valgus knee deformities.

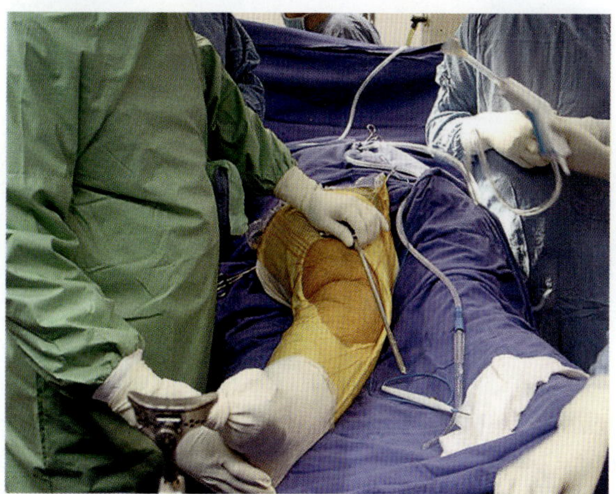

FIG. 3: Preoperative valgus deformity being demonstrated with alignment rod.

parapatellar approach is used). Identification of severity and correctability of the knee valgus is paramount before embarking on the surgical approach **(Fig. 4)**. During exposure, care must be taken not to compromise the medial soft tissue sleeve, which may already be attenuated. The lateral capsule is released from the tibia.

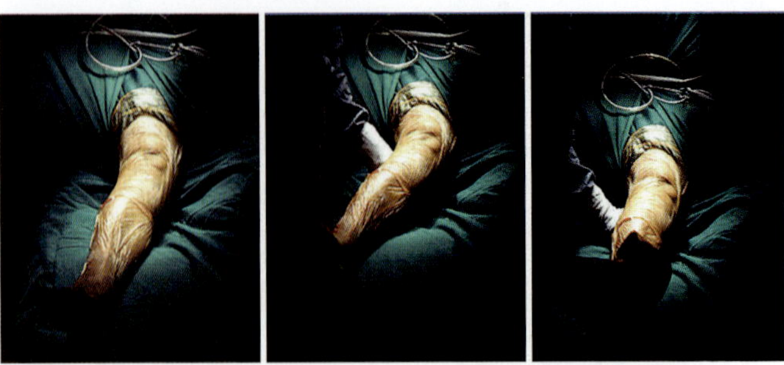

FIG. 4: Checking the severity and correctability of valgus deformity under anesthesia.

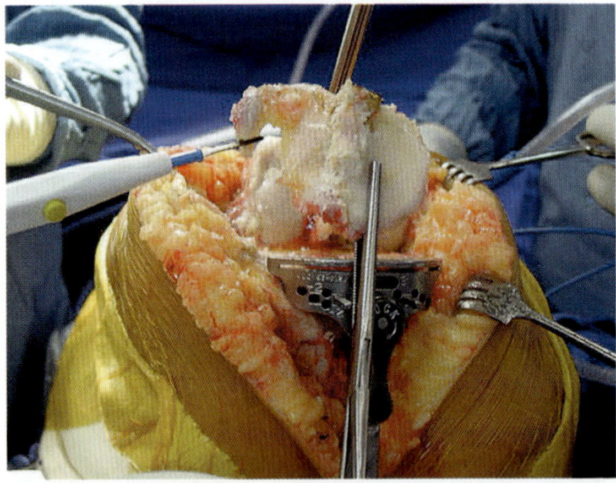

FIG. 5: Proximal tibial cut showing very little lateral tibial plateau bone excision.

- *Bone cuts*: The tibial cut is logically reverse to that of the varus knee, i.e., more bone is resected from medial side **(Fig. 5)**. Similarly, the lateral femoral condyle is more worn out (*or hypoplastic*) and must not be chased unnecessarily **(Fig. 6)**.
- *Soft tissue balancing*: Depending on the severity of deformity, an incremental release approach can be followed. First *release the anterior fibers of the iliotibial band* (selective release) from the Gerdy's tubercle, or alternatively at the level of the joint line. This can be done using the outside-in or the inside-out technique. Next, the anterior tibial musculature may be elevated from the anterolateral tibial surface. With greater fixed deformity, the lateral collateral ligament (LCL) is stripped off the lateral femoral

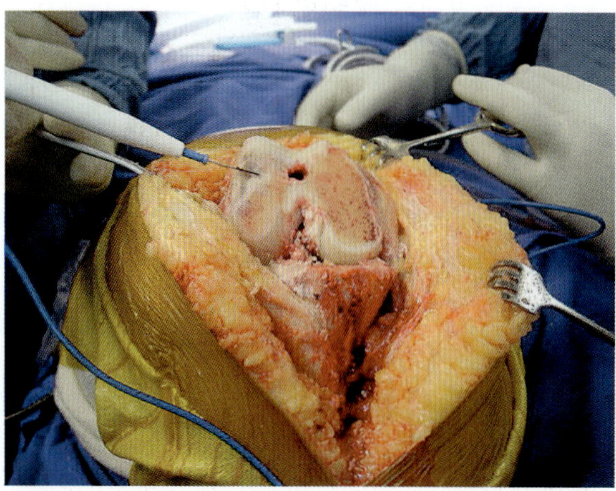

FIG. 6: Lateral femoral condyle defect seen after making distal femoral cut.

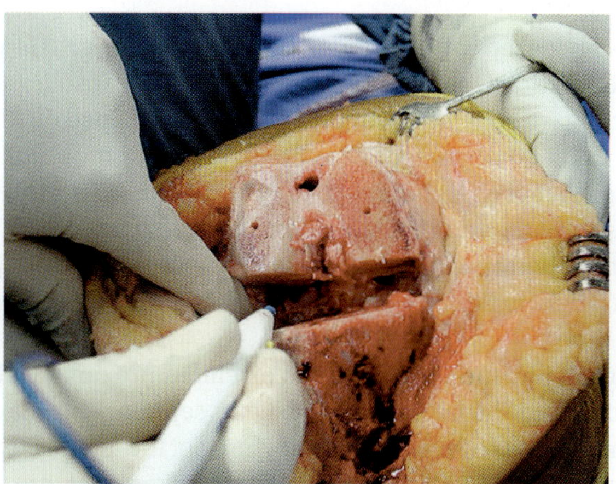

FIG. 7: Piecrust lengthening of posterolateral capsule.

condyle along with the popliteus tendon. If further release is needed, the periosteum of fibular head may be resected. Release or lengthening of the biceps femoris tendon is rarely performed.

If release is planned at the joint level (Ranawat technique), a titrated pie crust lengthening and/or release can be done of the LCL, popliteus, and posterolateral capsule **(Fig. 7)**. In very severe fixed valgus deformity, we can resort to lateral epicondyle sliding osteotomy. The posterior cruciate ligament (PCL) is almost always

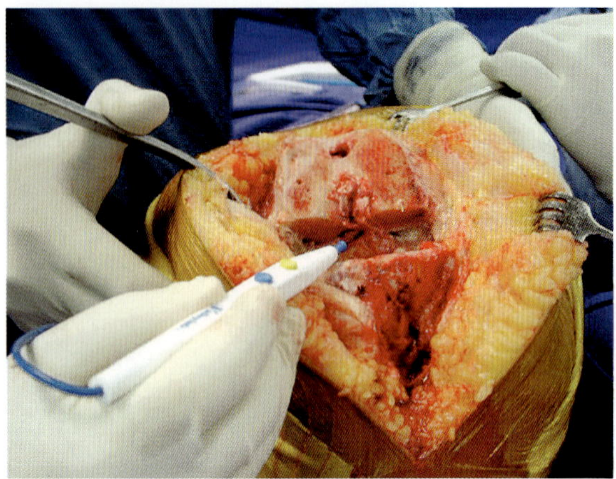

FIG. 8: Posterior cruciate ligament being cut with cautery.

sacrificed/released by the operating surgeon **(Fig. 8)**. With an associated flexion contracture, the posterolateral capsule and lateral head of the gastrocnemius may also need to be stripped off the femur.

The functional anatomic approach (Whiteside) utilizes the distinction between tightness in extension; tightness in flexion; or tightness in both, and thereafter focuses on release of the IT band and posterolateral capsule alone (tight in extension); or the LCL and popliteus (tight in flexion); or a titrated release of all lateral structures (tight in both).

Occasionally, the LCL release is extended proximally along the femur, lifting up the lateral intermuscular septum. This may lead to flexion instability with significant widening of the lateral flexion gap.

When combined valgus and flexion deformities are present, acute correction can cause stretching of the peroneal nerve and subsequent palsy.

In type II valgus knees, because of attenuation of the medial collateral ligament (MCL), adequate ligament balance cannot be obtained, and a constrained condylar type of prosthesis may be a reasonable option. The other option in this circumstance is MCL advancement, as described by Krackow, which includes elevation of the femoral origin of the MCL and proximal advancement using a locking-loop type of suture within the substance of the ligament. This suture is secured about a screw and washer with a staple placed in its desired attachment in the medial epicondyle.

The aim is to reach a mechanically well-aligned and balanced knee, with corrected deformities **(Figs. 9 to 11)**.

- *Patellofemoral tracking*: Patella usually lies laterally and may need lateral retinacular release **(Fig. 12)**. After release, the patellar tracking approximates the normal.
- Closure

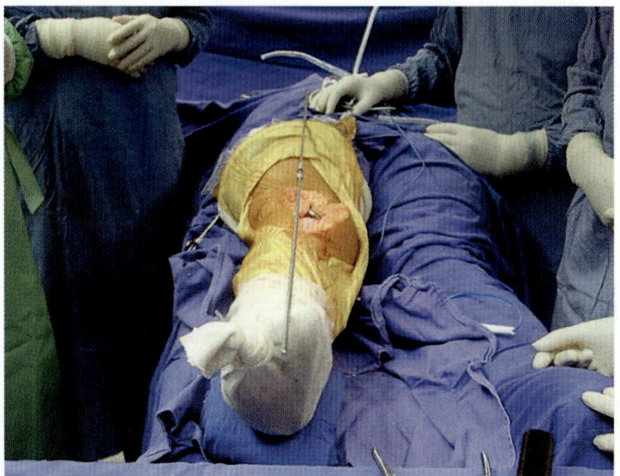

FIG. 9: Intraoperative achievement of correct alignment after release.

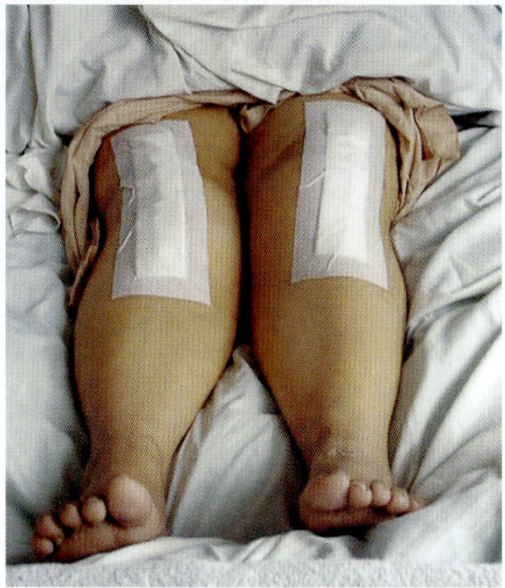

FIG. 10: Postoperative clinical photograph of corrected valgus deformities.

- *Special care*: Special care must be given to the lateral popliteal nerve, as the danger of stretching and causing paresis of the tibialis anterior and extensor hallucis longus (EHL) are very real.

In fixed valgus knees, a lateral parapatellar approach, with extensive lateral and posterolateral release (with/without fibula head excavation), and sometimes a lateral epicondyle sliding osteotomy, may be needed.

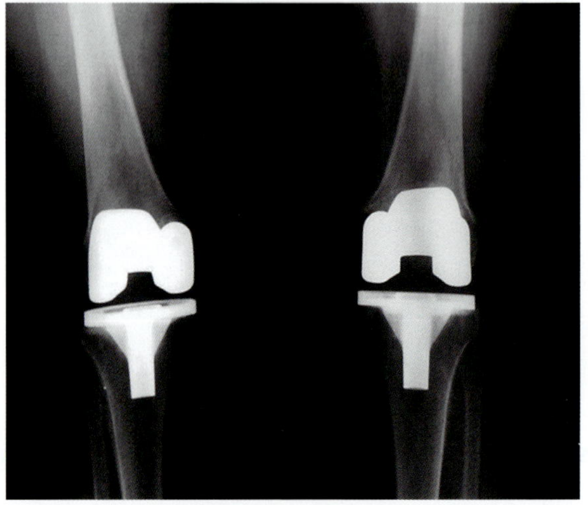

FIG. 11: Postoperative X-rays of corrected valgus deformities.

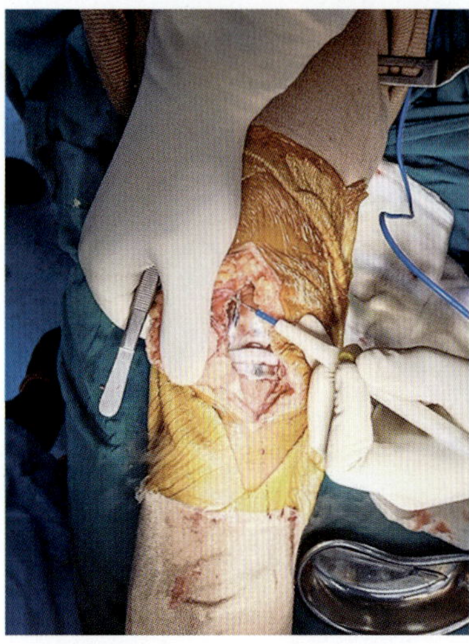

FIG. 12: Intraoperative picture showing inside-out lateral retinacular release.

Chapter 14

Surgical Technique: Flexion Deformity

As arthritis progresses, both varus and valgus knees may end up with an additional flexion deformity. Though the sequence of releases and correction for varus and valgus knees remain as decribed in the chapters on surgical technique of varus and valgus deformity, fixed flexion deformities pose special challenges **(Figs. 1 and 2)**.

- *Arthritic knee in flexion*:
  - Altered anatomical axis: Sagittal plane femoral and tibial axes are at an angle.
  - Altered biomechanical axis: It passes posterior to knee joint center. There may be associated varus/posterior tibial subluxation.
- *Patient position, incision, approach, and exposure*: With a fixed flexion contracture, the shortened posterior soft tissues block full extension.

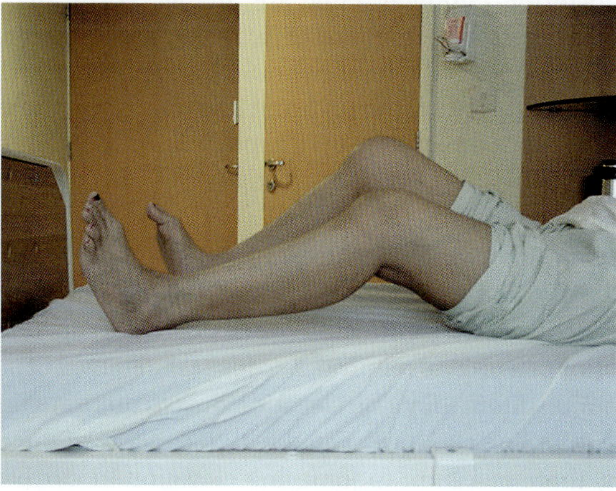

FIG. 1: Clinical photograph of patient with flexed knee deformities.

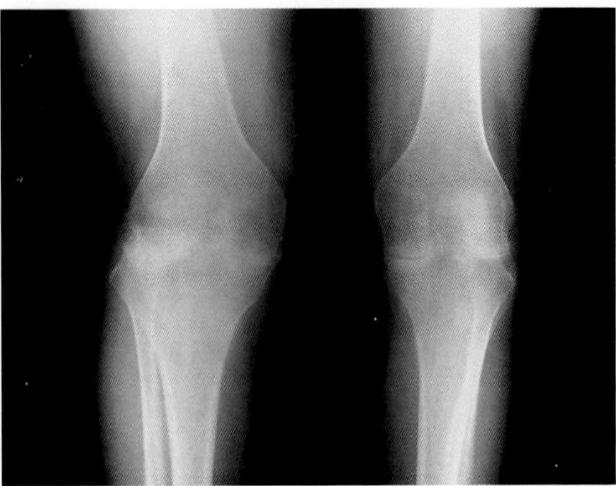

FIG. 2: X-rays of a typical patient with flexed knee deformities.

- *Bone cuts*: When excessive distal femoral resection is done to obtain extension, the knee may be stable in full extension because of a posterior tension band effect, but with slight flexion, the knee may lack varus-valgus stability. In this situation, the collateral ligaments are relatively longer than the posterior soft tissue restraints. A constrained condylar type of prosthesis may be necessary to resolve this "mid-flexion instability".
- *Soft tissue balancing*: The first step is to recreate the normal posterior capsular recesses of the knee joint by stripping the adherent posterior capsule proximally off the femur a short distance above the femoral condyles posteriorly, usually after the posterior condylar cuts are made. Posterior condylar osteophytes also are removed **(Fig. 3)**. Large osteophytes on the posterior aspect of the femur should be removed with a curved osteotome. The posterior capsule can be further released by stripping more proximally up the posterior aspect of the femur and releasing the tendinous origins of the gastrocnemius muscles if necessary.

Removing additional bone from the distal femur enlarges the narrowed extension gap **(Figs. 4 and 5)**. This should be used only with persistent flexion contracture after posterior capsular release and posterior osteophyte removal, because the removal of additional distal femur results in joint line elevation. Just as there is a limit to the extent the joint line can be elevated with balancing of the collateral ligaments, there is a limit to joint line elevation in correction of a severe flexion contracture, even with a posterior cruciate ligament

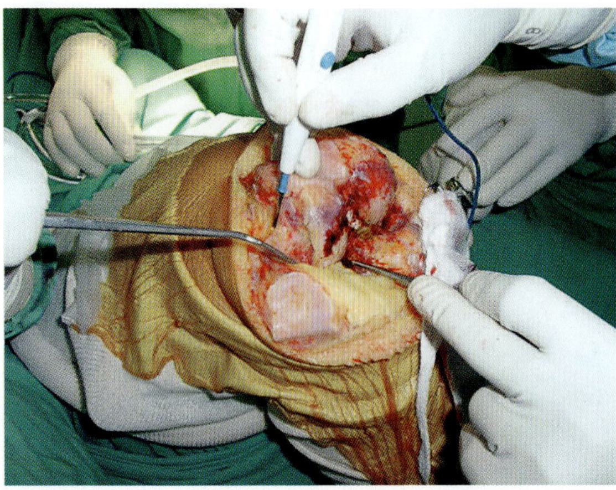

FIG. 3: Lateral parapatellar and lateral gutter release.

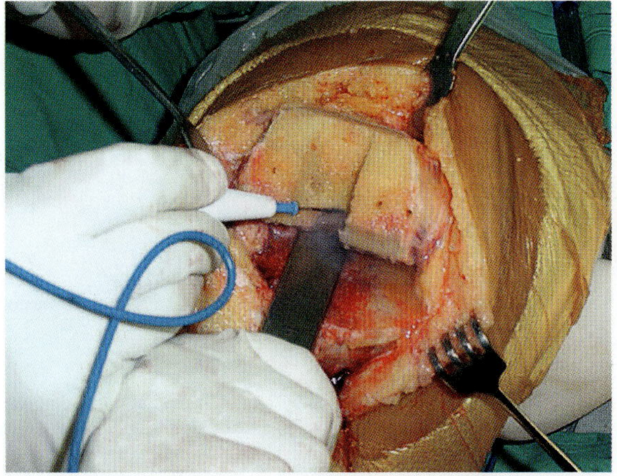

FIG. 4: Extensive posterior capsular release from posterior femur.

(PCL)-substituting prosthesis. Occasionally, the posterior capsule is also released off the posterior aspect of the proximal tibia **(Fig. 6)**.

- Patellar tracking, stability, and mobility
- *Closure*: Usually routine. However, if the flexion deformity is severe or associated with posterior subluxation of the tibia, expect difficulty in wound closure.
- *Special care*: Traction injury to the lateral popliteal nerve and posterior tibial vessels is a known complication that needs to be kept in mind.

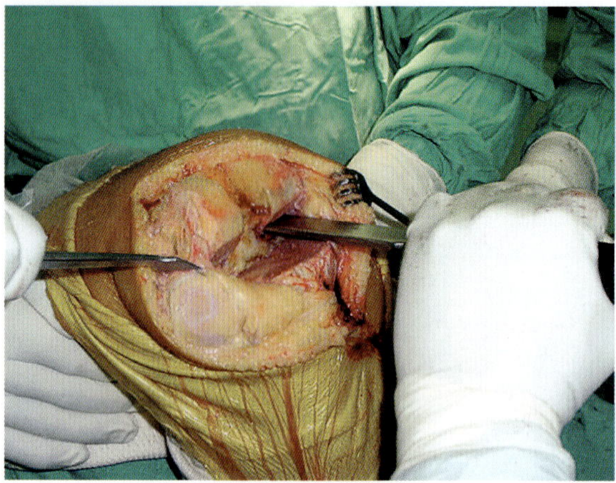

FIG. 5: Extensive release from posterior femoral condyles including removal of osteophytes.

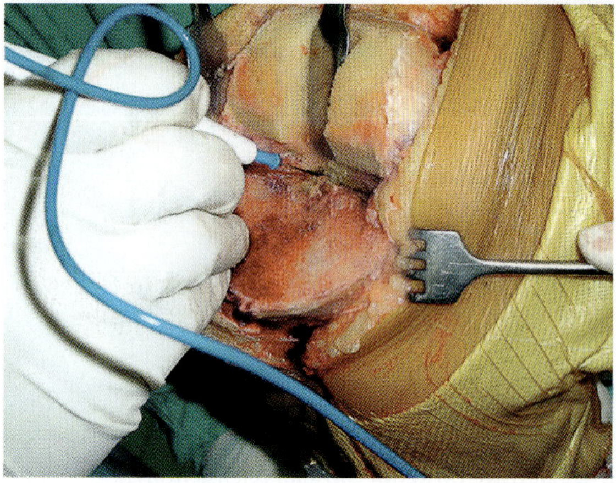

FIG. 6: Extensive posterior capsular release from posterior tibia.

- Even if we have adequately released the posterior structures and achieved complete extension intraoperatively **(Figs. 7 and 8)**, it may be a good idea to keep the knee flexed to 20–30° postoperatively for 2–3 days and gradually extend it to minimize the chances of neural damage. The knee will gradually correct to full extension with time once the pain and inflammation subside.

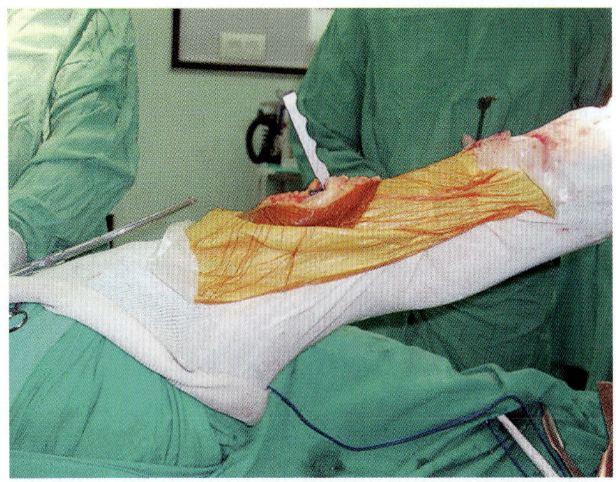

FIG. 7: Knee position after correction of flexion deformity.

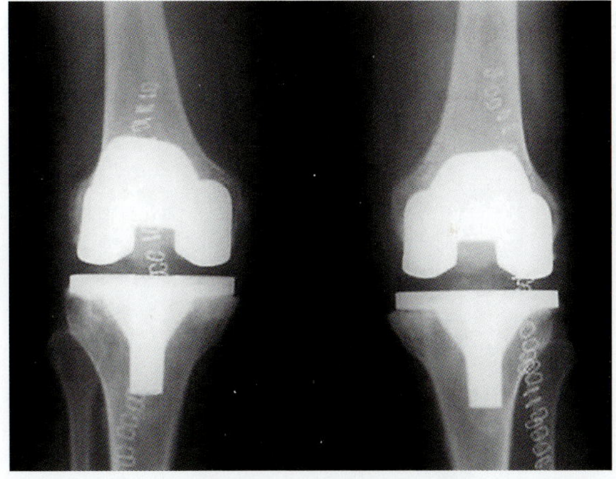

FIG. 8: Postoperative X-rays of corrected flexed knee deformities.

Chapter 15

Surgical Technique: Bone Defect Management

Bone deficiencies encountered can have multiple causes, including arthritic angular deformity, condylar hypoplasia, avascular necrosis, trauma, and previous surgery such as high tibial osteotomy and previous total knee replacement. The method used to compensate for a given bone defect depends on both the size and location of the defect **(Figs. 1 and 2)**.

Contained or cavitary defects have an intact rim of cortical bone surrounding the deficient area, whereas uncontained or segmental defects are more peripheral and lack a bony cortical rim.

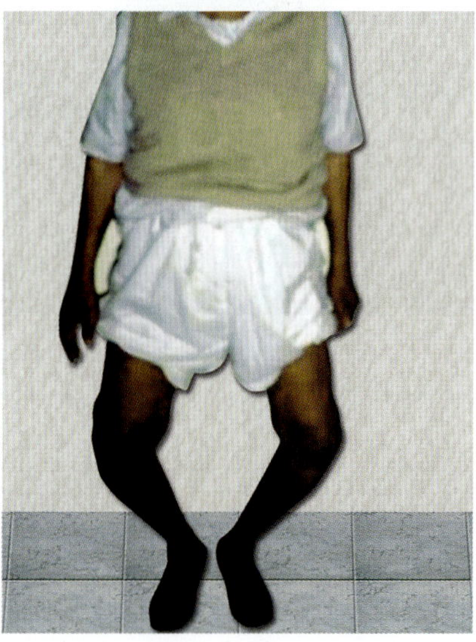

FIG. 1: Clinical photograph of patient with bone defects (severe varus knees).

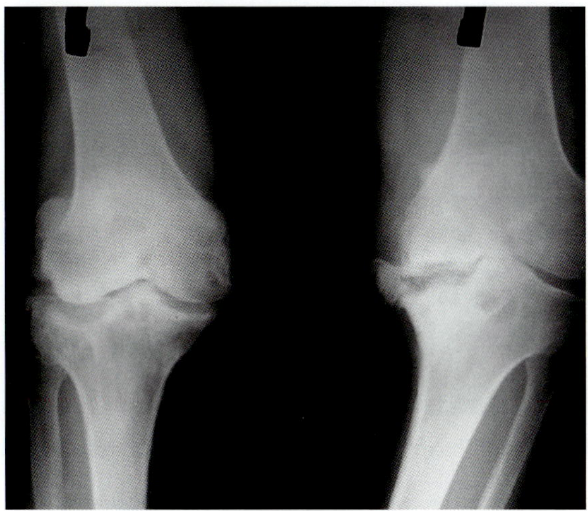

FIG. 2: X-rays of a typical patient with bone defects (severe varus knees).

Rand has classified these defects into three types:

- *Type I:* Focal metaphyseal defect and intact cortical rim.
- *Type II:* Extensive metaphyseal defect and intact cortical rim.
- *Type III:* Combined metaphyseal and cortical defect.

SPECIAL CARE

Small defects (<5 mm) typically are filled with cement **(Figs. 3 and 4)**. Contained defects can also be filled with impacted cancellous bone graft **(Figs. 5 and 6)**. Larger uncontained defects (more than 5 mm) can be treated by a variety of methods, including structural bone grafts, metal wedges, or blocks attached to the prostheses or screws within cement that fills the defect. The technique remains an option, especially in older patients.

Multiple techniques for bone grafting of peripheral defects of the tibia have been described. Windsor, Insall, and Sculco convert the concave, irregular defect to a flat one by minimal bone removal with a saw. Bone removed from the distal femur or proximal tibia is attached to the flattened defect and secured with screws. The upper tibial surface is then carefully recut to create a flat upper tibial surface. Occasionally, irregular bone ridges should be leveled with a burr to allow maximal graft-host bone apposition. The graft then can be fashioned to fit the defect **(Fig. 7)**. This can also be done using metal augments **(Fig. 8)**. Rand reported the results of cemented tibial wedges in 28 knees.

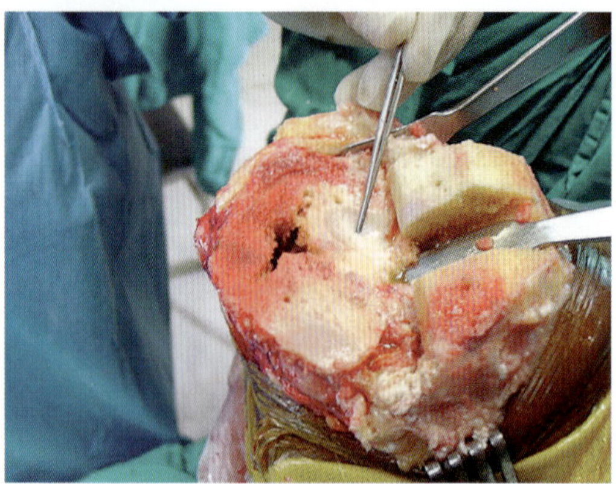

FIG. 3: Minor (<5 mm depth) contained defect in tibial plateau.

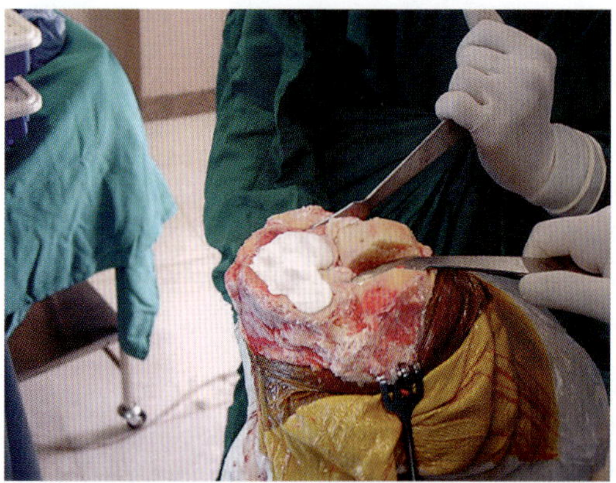

FIG. 4: Defect managed with bone cement.

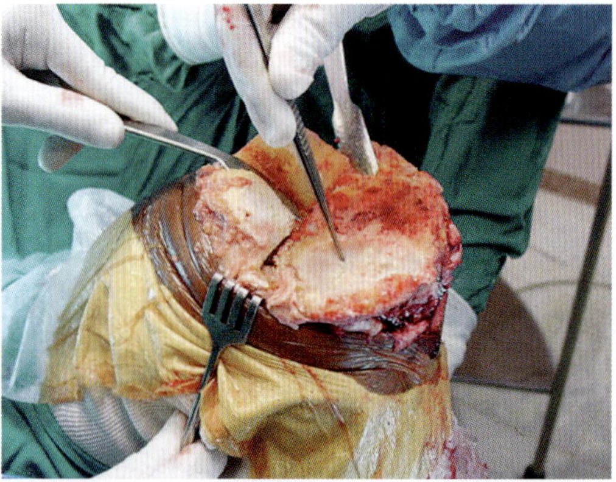

FIG. 5: Major (>5 mm depth) contained defect in tibial plateau.

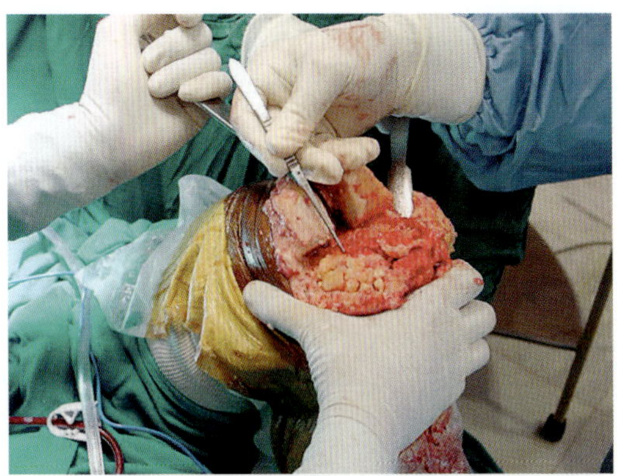

FIG. 6: Defect managed with morselized impaction bone grafting.

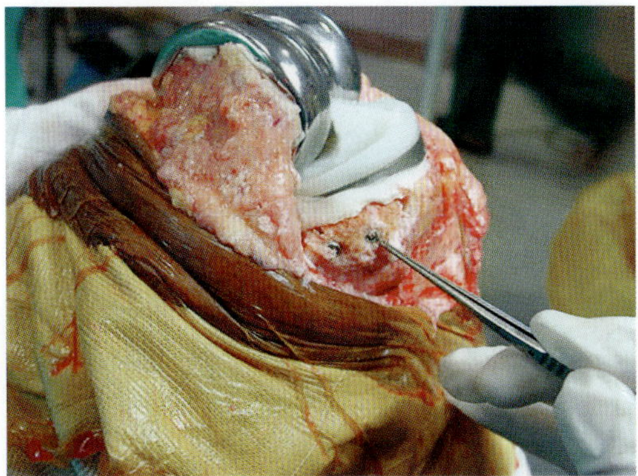

FIG. 7: Uncontained major bone defect in tibial plateau managed with strut grafting and fixation with screws.

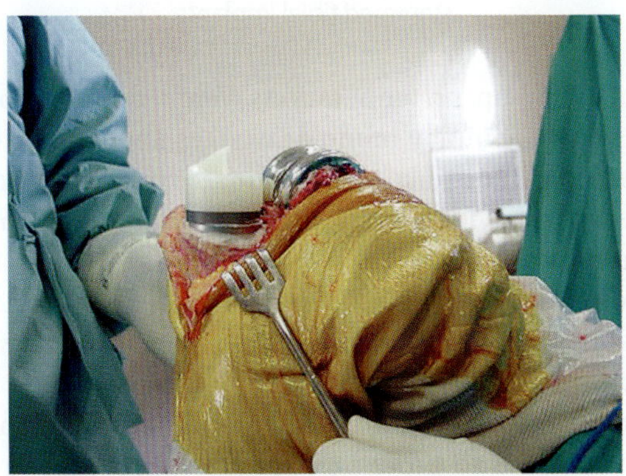

FIG. 8: Uncontained major bone defect in tibial plateau managed with metal wedge.

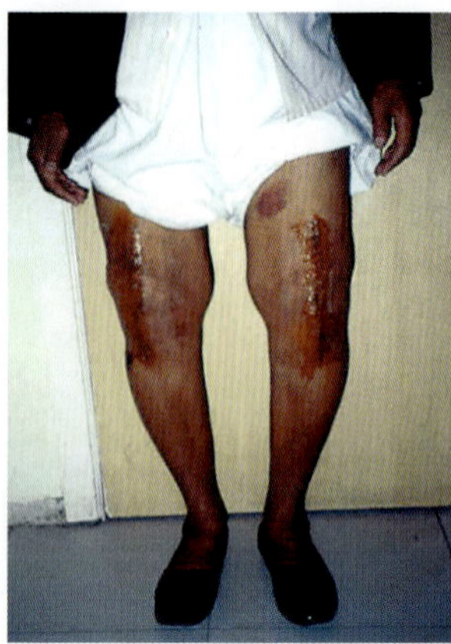

FIG. 9: Postoperative clinical photograph of patient with grafted bone defects.

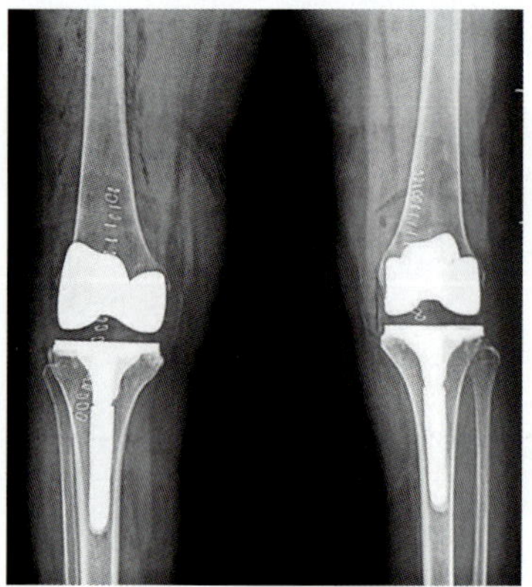

FIG. 10: Postoperative X-rays of patient with impacted bone grafts and stemmed tibial implants.

At 2.3 years follow-up, no reoperations were required. Most modern total knee systems employ modular wedges and blocks that can be attached to femoral and tibial components to compensate for multiple bone deficiencies. With these structural additions, a surgeon can literally build a custom prosthesis in the operating room for a given defect or combination of defects.

Restoration of neutral alignment is essential because this has been shown to affect bone graft survival and prosthesis loosening. Intramedullary stems on both the femoral and tibial components commonly are used to protect peripheral bone grafts from stress. With the use of intramedullary stems to bypass the defects, good long-term results have been universally shown **(Figs. 9 and 10)**.

Chapter 16

Surgical Technique: Recurvatum Deformity

Recurvatum deformity is unusual and can pose significant surgical challenges. The cause of the recurvatum (whether due to muscle imbalances, or gradually progressive bony erosion) must be clarified, as results can be universally poor if the prosthetic knee is left in hyperextension (>5°). Since the advent of computer-assisted and robotic-assisted surgery, genu recurvatum has been found to be more prevalent (4–12%). The main causes of this deformity include neuromuscular disorders, rheumatoid arthritis, inverted tibial slope, or conditions associated with coronal deformities such as genu valgum **(Figs. 1 to 3)**. Quadriceps weakness or paralysis may

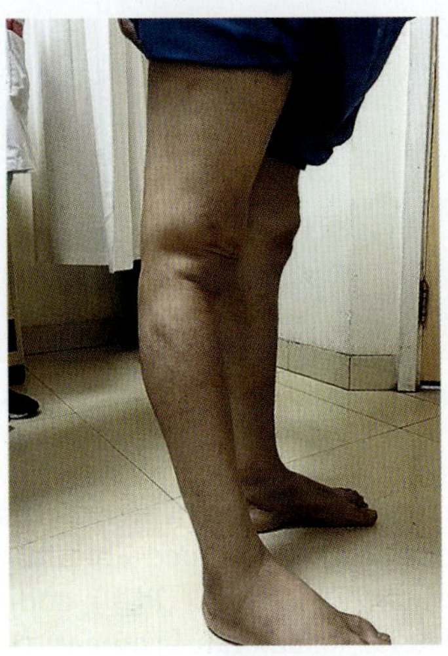

FIG. 1: Preoperative clinical photograph of patient with recurvatum right knee deformity.

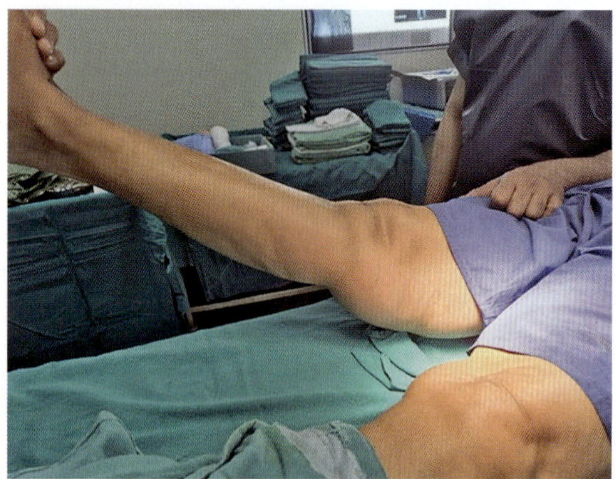

FIG. 2: Patient with recurvatum right knee deformity under anesthesia.

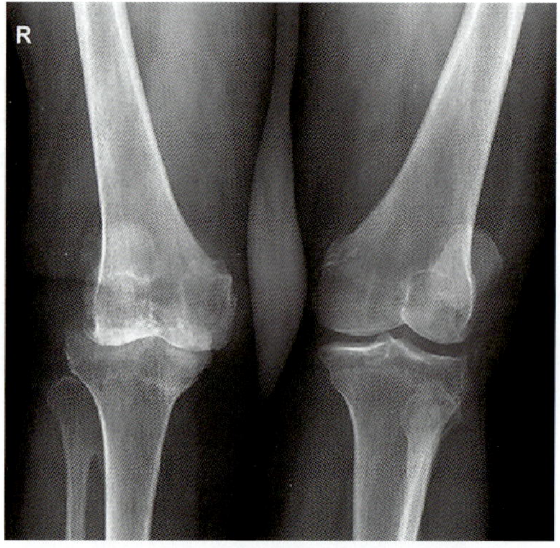

FIG. 3: X-rays of the patient with recurvatum right knee deformity.

lead the patient to lock the knee in hyperextension during gait as a compensatory mechanism. Combined anterior cruciate ligament (ACL)/posterior cruciate ligament (PCL) and medial collateral ligament (MCL)/lateral collateral ligament (LCL) laxity could predispose to prosthetic instability.

- *Arthritic knee in recurvatum*:
    - Altered anatomical axis: Sagittal plane femoral and tibial axes are at an angle.
    - Altered biomechanical axis: It passes anterior to knee joint center. There may be associated varus/anterior tibial subluxation.
- *Patient position, incision, approach, and exposure*: In a recurvatum deformity, the lengthened posterior soft tissues with/without defects in the anterior bone of the femur and tibia lead to hyperextension. Position, incision, and approach remain the same.
- *Bone cuts*: The goal is to create an extension gap that is a symmetrical rectangle of equal size and shape to the flexion gap. The go-to method in recurvatum deformity is to take minimal femoral and tibial cuts. The tibial cut is usually taken either flush with the worn-out surface (medial plateau) or just 2 mm off it. The distal femoral cut is taken 2–4 mm less than the standard cut using the jig **(Fig. 4)**. A standard (or slightly larger) spacer provides stable extension balance after these minimal cuts.

  Anterior referencing is done for the femur, and the largest size of the femur that provides a stable flexion gap (without tightness/contracture) is chosen, and cuts taken accordingly **(Fig. 5)**.
- *Soft tissue balancing*: The first step is to recreate the normal posterior slope of the proximal tibia (as many times recurvatum is associated with a reverse tibial slope). No posterior/medial/lateral release is attempted, unless associated varus/valgus dictate otherwise.

Another approach to achieve gap symmetry is the gap balancing technique, where the proximal tibia is initially cut at 90° of its mechanical axis. Subsequently, with the knee flexed to 90° and considering medial and lateral ligament tension, the distal femur and posterior femur are resected to achieve appropriate external rotation of the femoral component, thus equalizing both gaps and achieving full extension without recurvatum **(Fig. 6)**.

- *Patellar tracking, stability, and mobility*: It is important to note that the joint line should not be modified more than 4 mm proximally or distally to avoid instability in the midrange of flexion (mid-flexion instability).
- *Closure*: Usually routine

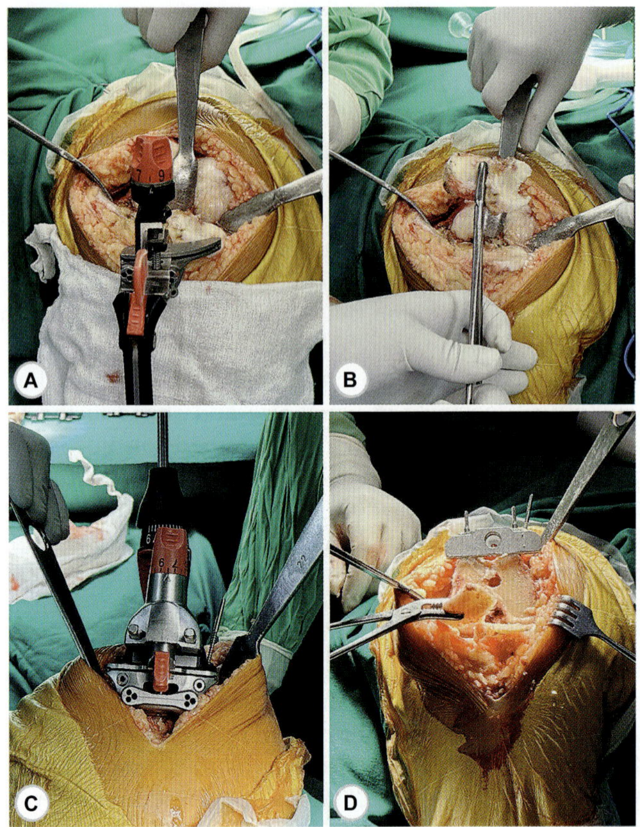

FIGS. 4 A TO D: Intraoperative photos showing minimal tibial and femoral cuts to identify extension gap.

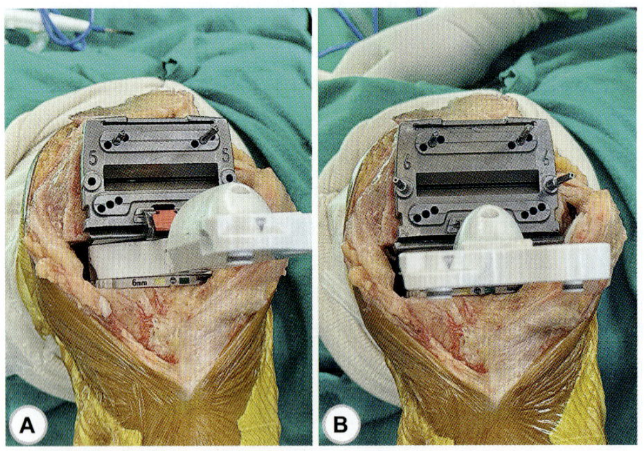

FIGS. 5 A AND B: Intraoperative photos showing use of large femoral size to balance gaps.

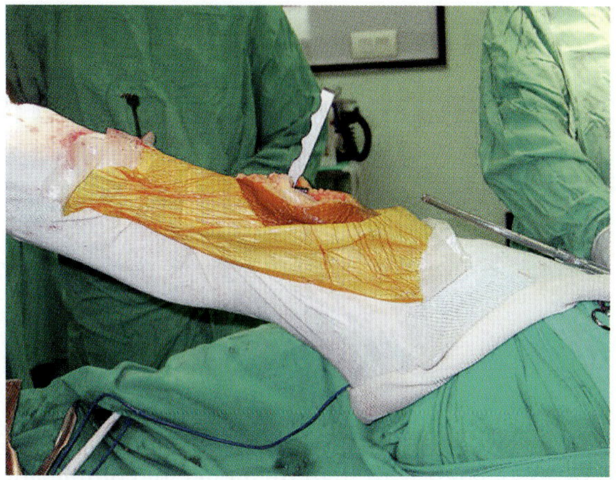

FIG. 6: Knee position after correction of recurvatum deformity.

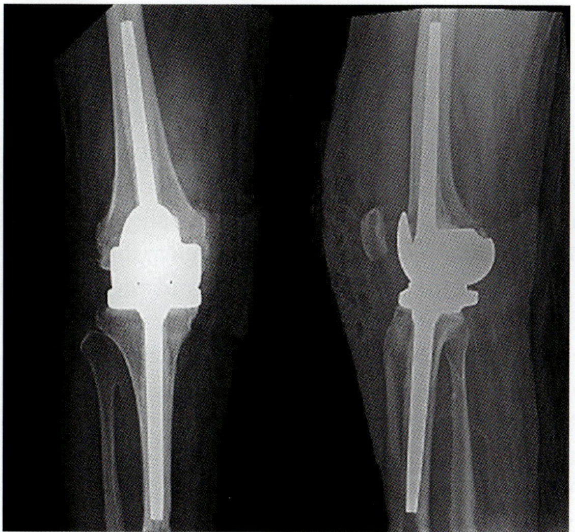

FIG. 7: Postoperative X-rays of corrected recurvatum knee deformities wherein rotating hinged implants were used.

- *Special care*: The primary complication associated with this population is the recurrence of the recurvatum deformity due to ligamentous and soft-tissue hypermobility. Constrained knees with rotating hinges must be used in these cases **(Fig. 7)**.

Chapter 17

Surgical Technique: Fused Knee Takedown

Fused (ankylosed) knees pose excessive challenges and have shown to be associated with high incidence of complications such as knee stiffness, extensor mechanism insufficiency, instability, implant failure, and periprosthetic joint infection. Prerequisites for patients undergoing this procedure are a sufficient extensor mechanism and adequate soft-tissue coverage. In addition, realistic patient expectations with regards to the functional outcome, meticulous planning, and willingness and motivation of the patient to continuously participate in the postoperative follow-up care are imperative for success of this uncommon procedure.

Previously operated knees (arthrodesed/infected TKAs) undergoing intramedullary fusion are a different ball game and need even more soft tissue care and attention to surgical discipline to prevent wound healing and recurrent stiffness, and these have not been discussed here. A thorough patient selection process thus aids in the positive outcome of this rare procedure **(Fig. 1)**.

- *Arthrodesed/fused knee*:
  - Altered anatomical axis: Depends on the position of fusion, and so, needs attention
  - Altered biomechanical axis: Depends on the underlying pathology preceding fusion, or the previous underlying injury/surgery leading to arthrodesis
  - Joint line: The meniscal scar remains as a marker for joint line position (in pathological conditions that lead to ankylosis). However, in previously operated cases, this may not apply.

Other issues include the availability of very little skin and soft tissues (previously operated/arthrodesed knees), inability to assess ligaments [medial collateral ligament (MCL)/lateral collateral

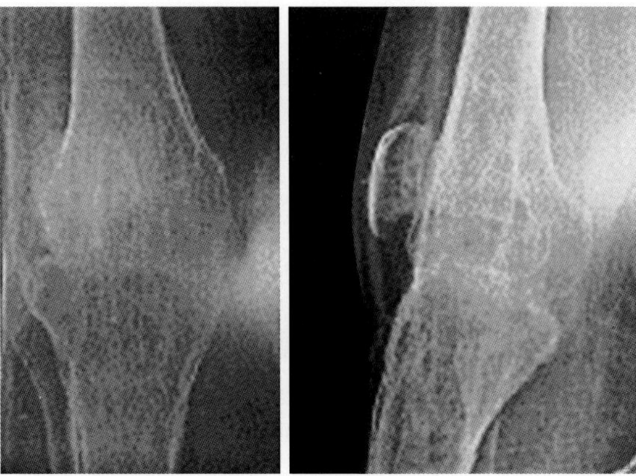

FIG. 1: X-rays of a patient with fused knee planned for conversion to TKA.

ligament (LCL)], soft osteoporotic bones, and quadriceps shortening (because of the long-standing knee position).

- *Patient position, incision, approach, and exposure*: Supine position, incision (along previous scar, if present) is extended proximally and distally, and the skin/subcutaneous tissue undermined in one layer to develop sleeves (for closure), occasionally skin expanders are used 2–3 months prior to the planned surgery (to prevent wound closure problems). Extended medial parapatellar approach (with redevelopment of medial and lateral gutters) and re-establishment of the patellofemoral space (with an oscillating screw/osteotome) all the way up to the mid-thigh are almost always essential. Occasionally, a tibial tubercle osteotomy approach with pie-crust lengthening of the quadriceps or a V-Y quadricepsplasty may be needed. Adequate exposure is the key **(Fig. 2)**.
- *Bone cuts*: Initially the joint line level is assessed (using meniscal scar/fibular head/medial and lateral femoral epicondyles/image intensifier) and an 8–10 mm block of bone removed around this level (double osteotomy). Care must be taken to stop just short of the posterior cortex and manipulation used to complete the osteotomies, as the posterior neurovascular structures lie just behind the capsule **(Fig. 3)**. Gradual knee flexion will be possible after removal of this osteotomy block. The definitive tibial cut is then taken using appropriate bony landmarks and image intensifier **(Fig. 4)**.

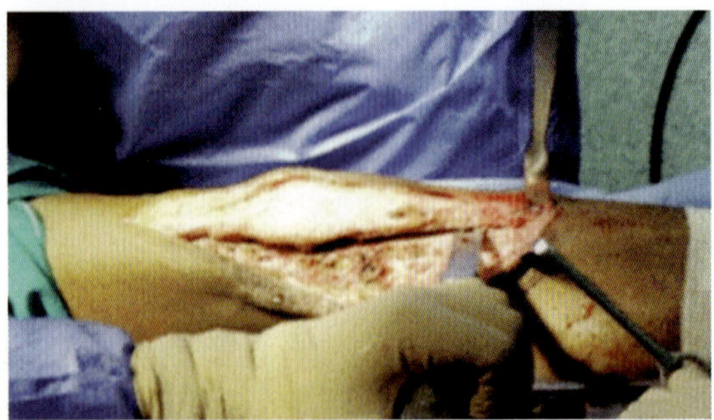

FIG. 2: Intraoperative picture showing patellofemoral space creation with osteotomy extending to include tibial tubercle.

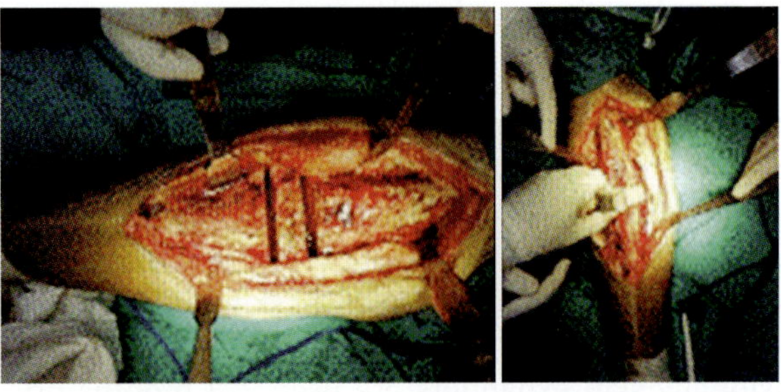

FIG. 3: Intraoperative picture showing double level osteotomy at joint line.

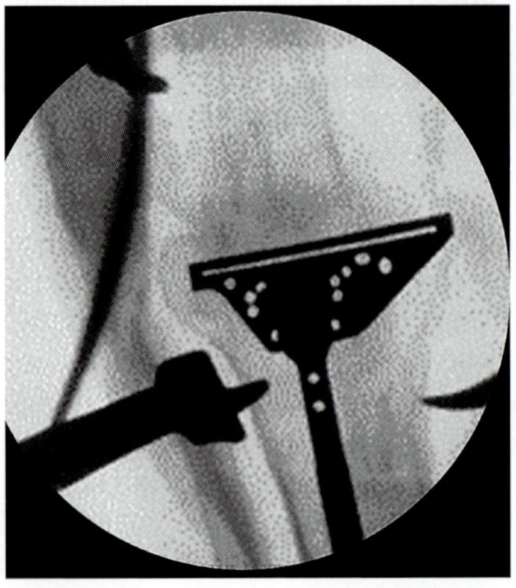

FIG. 4: Intraoperative picture showing tibial jig placement using image intensifier.

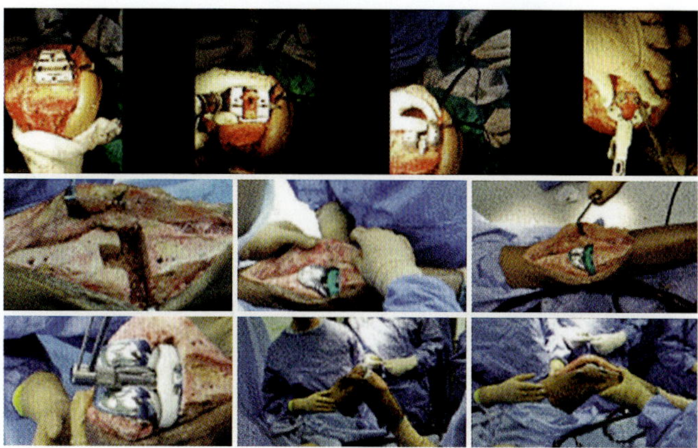

FIG. 5: Intraoperative pictures showing femoral jig placement in flexion.

Anterior referencing is done for the femur, and the smallest size of the femur that provides a stable flexion gap (without anterior notching/contracture) is chosen, and cuts taken accordingly **(Figs. 3 and 5)**.

- *Soft tissue balancing*: MCL and LCL are checked for integrity and stability, and if inadequate, provision made for a rotating hinged prosthesis. Flexion range is examined and a V-Y quadricepsplasty performed (to lengthen the tight quadriceps and permit knee flexion).

It is important to note that the joint line should not be modified more than 4 mm proximally or distally to avoid instability in the midrange of flexion (mid-flexion instability).

Another approach to achieve gap symmetry is the gap balancing technique, where the proximal tibia is initially cut at 90° to its mechanical axis. Subsequently, with the knee flexed to 90° and considering medial and lateral ligament tension, the distal femur and posterior femur are resected to achieve appropriate external rotation of the femoral component, thus equalizing both gaps.

- Patellar tracking, stability, and mobility
- *Closure*: An inverted V incision taken at the musculotendinous junction of the quadriceps is sutured in Y-shape with the knee flexed to 45–50°. Tibial tubercle osteotomy is fixed with two screws. Wound is closed in anatomical layers and the knee supported by a graduated hinged knee brace adjusted to keep the knee in full extension for the first 48 hours.

Gradually progressive continuous passive motion (CPM)/knee bending (limited to 30° for the first 3 weeks), and then to maximum

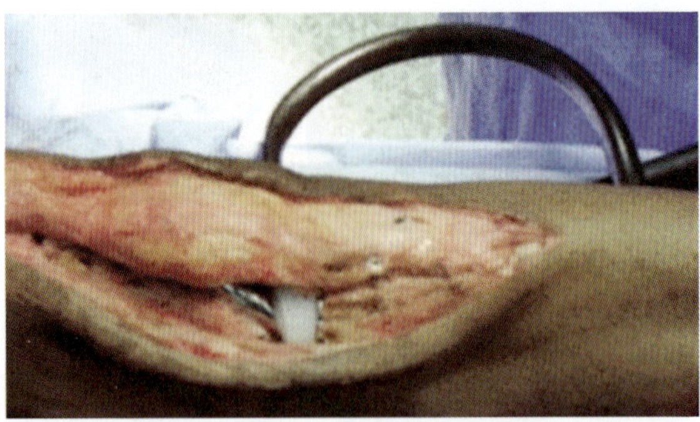

FIG. 6: Postoperative picture after V-Y quadricepsplasty and tibial tubercle osteotomy fixation.

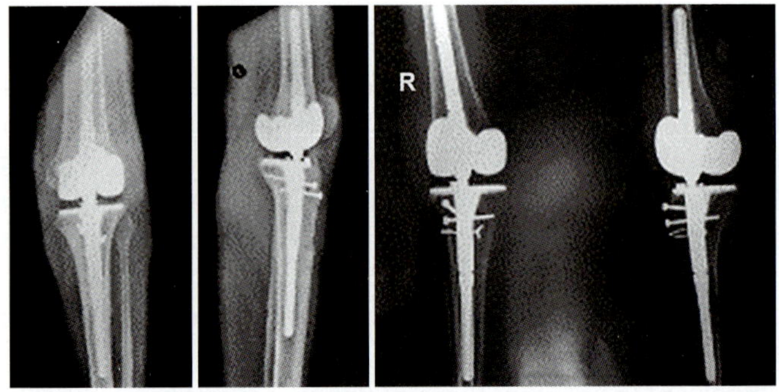

FIG. 7: Postoperative X-rays of knee after fusion take down.

permitted is allowed and encouraged, as well as full weight bearing walking. Quadriceps strengthening exercises are initiated at 6–8 weeks.

- *Special care*: If the MCL/LCL are compromised during surgery (especially in completely ankylosed knees), a rotating hinged knee prosthesis is inserted with femoral and tibial stems **(Figs. 6 and 7)**.

Chapter 18

Postoperative Period

TRANSPORTATION TO THE RECOVERY ROOM

- Supine with leg supported over two pillows, no need for bracing
- Cardiac monitoring and O_2 supplementation to accompany
- Patient should be catheterized (urinary) if undergoing simultaneous bilateral knee replacement, or in heavy female patients, and male patients with history of benign prostatic hypotrophy (BPH)

POSITION IN THE RECOVERY ROOM (FIG. 1)

- Continuous monitoring of heart rate, blood pressure (BP), respiratory rate (RR), electrocardiogram (ECG), and oxygen saturation (SpO_2) for the first 4 hours (or longer if indicated)

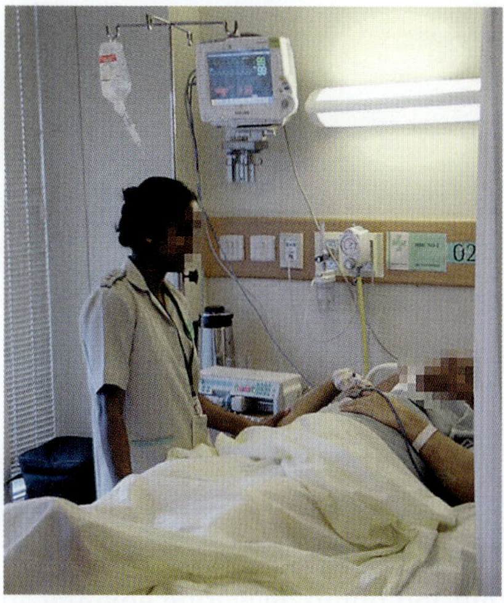

FIG. 1: Postoperative patient in recovery room.

- O_2 by face mask/ventimask/nasal prongs
- Antibiotic cover for gram positive and gram negative (usually cefuroxime ± amikacin, alternatively augmentin ± tobramycin)
- Blood transfusion to be started in the recovery
- Suction drains (if used) to be clamped for an hour, monitor and look out for local soakage (if any), and drain output and urine output
- Subcutaneous low-molecular-weight heparin (LMWH) to be started—body weight to be considered—about 8–10 hours postoperatively
- Distal neurovascular status to be checked (assess recovery from regional anesthesia)
- Regular pain assessment

PAIN MANAGEMENT

- *Pain control*: Epidural infusion/patient-controlled analgesia (PCA)/injectable analgesic. *It is easier to prevent pain than to chase pain* **(Fig. 2)**.
- The patient may be allowed turning in bed with a pillow between the knees.
- Cryotherapy (ice packs) locally
- Oral sips of clear fluid 2–3 hours postoperatively, followed by semisolids

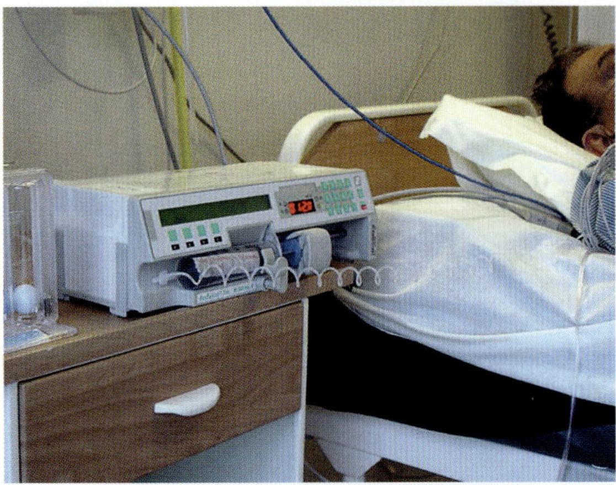

Fig. 2: Infusion pump delivering epidural analgesia.

- Encourage turning in bed with assistance by the evening... *prevent bedsores*. Sitting up may be permitted after anesthetist clearance.

IN THE WARDS: DAY 1

- Vitals to be monitored 4 hourly. O_2 supplementation if required. Drains to be removed.
- Hemoglobin (Hb)/packed cell volume (PCV) in the morning (others as required: sugars in diabetics, 12-lead ECG in cardiac patients, serum creatinine and serum electrolytes in renal compromised patients)
- Measurement of total drain output *(need for additional blood transfusion)*
- *Check all lines*: Foley's catheter, epidural catheter, and IV lines
- Check X-rays (portable)
- Compression stockings [mechanical deep vein thrombosis (DVT) prophylaxis] **(Fig. 3)** along with LMW heparin (chemoprophylaxis) to continue
- Physician to review for associated medication (insulin, antihypertensive, etc.)
- Epidural analgesia/PCA to continue
- Start physiotherapy (sitting up, standing, walking with walker support, and toilet training) **(Fig. 4)**

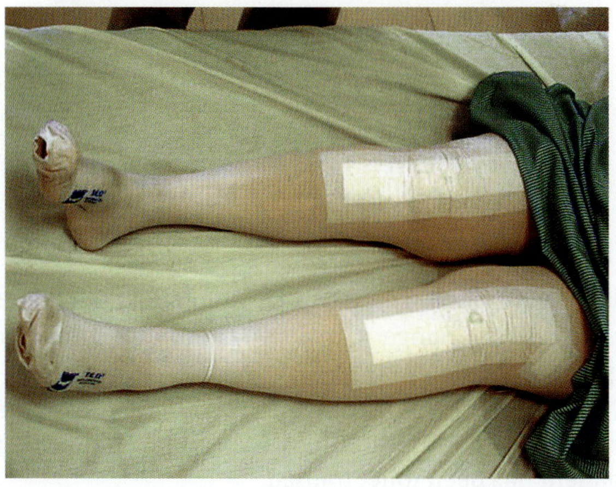

FIG. 3: Stockings for deep vein thrombosis (DVT) prophylaxis.

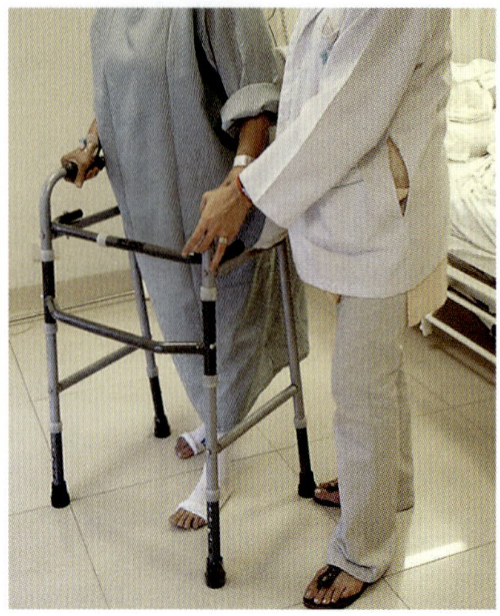

FIG. 4: Walking with walker.

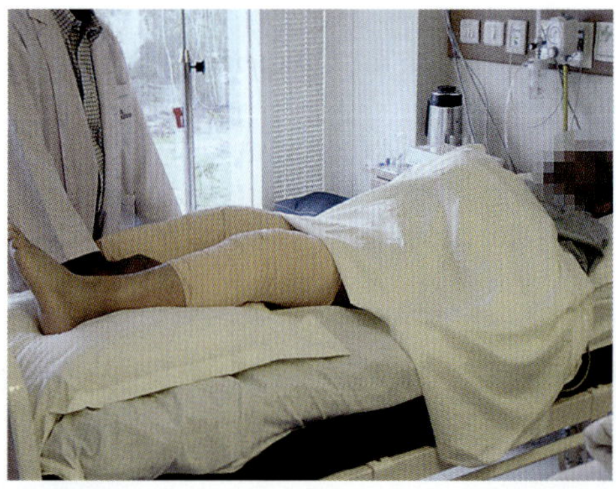

FIG. 5: Dressing after drain removal.

IN THE WARDS: DAY 2

- Vitals to be monitored 4 hourly. O_2 supplementation if required
- *Dressing check*: Change if soaked/soiled, else remove outer RJ compression bandages **(Fig. 5)**.
- Aim to remove Foley's catheter on this day, either morning (if unilateral), or by the afternoon (if bilateral), after ensuring that the patient has been toilet trained
- *Check remaining lines*: Epidural catheter and IV lines

- Compression stockings (mechanical DVT prophylaxis) along with LMW heparin (chemoprophylaxis) to continue
- Physician to review for associated medication (insulin, antihypertensive, etc.)
- Epidural analgesia/PCA to be reduced
- IV medication to be stopped, switched to oral meds
- Continue physiotherapy (sitting up, standing, walking with walker support, and toilet training) twice a day, progress to independent assisted ambulation in the corridor

MONITORING IN SPECIAL SITUATIONS

- Blood sugars in diabetics
- 12-lead ECG in cardiac patients
- Serum creatinine and serum electrolytes in renal compromised patients
- Measurement of total drain output *(need for additional blood transfusion).*

DISCHARGE CRITERIA

- Off all IV support (on oral meds—including medicine-related meds)
- Pain tolerated well with oral meds (off epidural/PCA/other parenteral analgesics)
- Ambulating well (standing and walking with support of walker)
- Bowels cleared (passed stools) or confirmed bowel movements

RED FLAGS

- Respiratory distress/drop in SpO_2 levels
- Drowsiness/drop in alertness level
- Consistent/persistent/recurrent fever
- Excessive local pain and inflammation
- Soakage *(change of entire dressing)*

Chapter 19

Accelerated Physiotherapy Protocol

We now follow an accelerated physiotherapy protocol that aims to get the patient back on his/her feet as well as back to his/her vocation at the earliest, at the same time ensuring safety. This accelerated protocol relies on adequate patient education and training (*prehabilitation*) before the surgery and regular feedback provided to the patient detailing his/her recovery. The exercises are standardized to include:

- *Quadriceps strengthening (and stretching):* Static and dynamic quadriceps exercises are ideally started preoperatively itself as they form a baseline on which postoperative mobilization and recovery depend. These are continued from the first day **(Fig. 1)**.

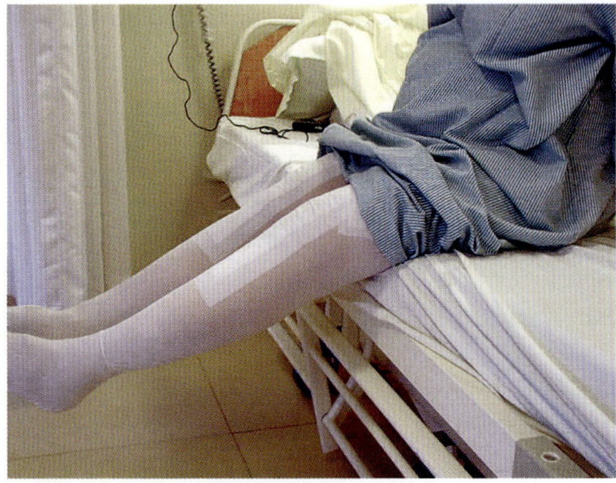

FIG. 1: Quadriceps setting exercises.

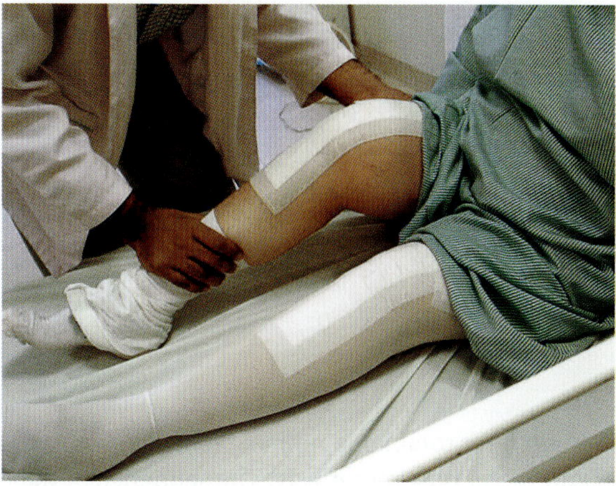

FIG. 2: Knee bending protocol.

- *Hamstring strengthening and stretching (knee bending):* Knee bending is gradually introduced from the second postoperative day, initially 30–40° and to 90° by the day of discharge **(Fig. 2)**.
- *Walking with walker aided support:* Started from the evening of surgery (in unilateral cases) and the morning after surgery (in bilateral cases). Usually, the elderly patient needs a walker for support and balance for up to 2–3 weeks, but in younger patients, the need for a walker is less.
- *Hip abductor and iliopsoas strengthening:* Hip muscle weakness plays a significant role in lurch and waddling gait in patients with severe knee arthritis. Hip strengthening exercises are initiated for improving gait as well as limb control during walking, change of position, and turning in bed.
- *Stick aided walking:* Once the patient has developed balance and gait control (2–3 weeks), he/she is encouraged to walk with a cane on the side opposite the operated limb (in unilateral cases) and on the stronger side (in bilateral cases) so that he/she gains confidence in independent ambulation.
- *Toilet training:* Toilet training using a high toilet seat is usually achieved by the second or third postoperative day and is one of the criteria for discharge.
- *Stair climbing (latest by 3 weeks):* Most patients with good quadriceps strength can climb a few stairs by the time they are discharged and encouraged to keep building on their quadriceps, hamstring, and hip muscle strengths.

Chapter 20

Follow-up

Usual follow-up after total knee replacement is at 2 weeks, 6 weeks, 3 months, and 1-year postoperatively. The sequence of major events following *unilateral* knee replacement consists of:

- Suture removal at 2–3 weeks (3 weeks in patients of rheumatoid arthritis) **(Fig. 1)**
- Walker aided ambulation for 1–2 weeks → walking stick/cane for another 1–2 weeks → independent ambulation (by 3–4 weeks)
- Stair climbing at 1–2 weeks
- Car driving at 3 months

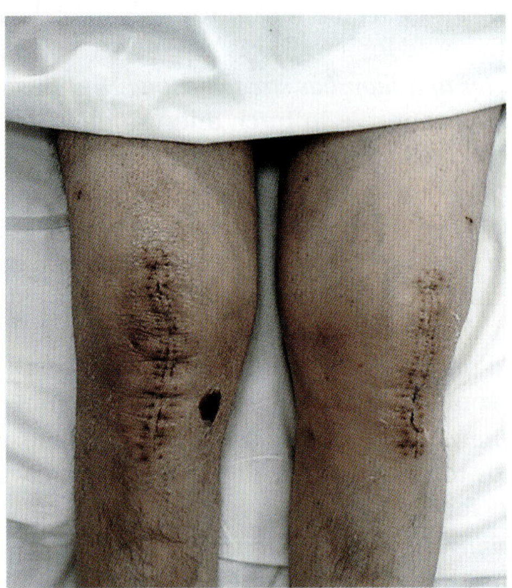

FIG. 1: At staple removal.

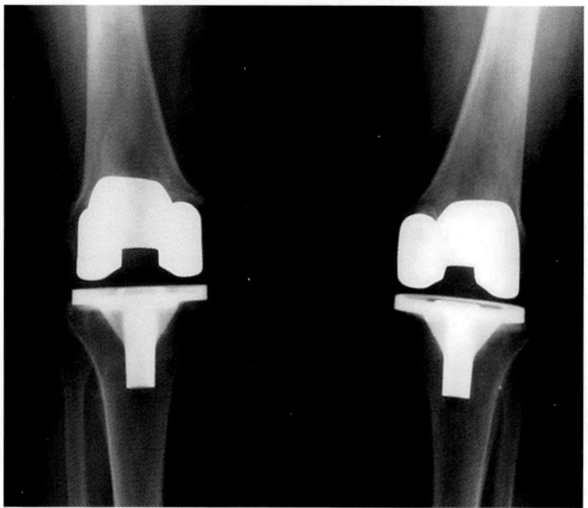

FIG. 2: X-rays at 3 months follow-up.

Following *bilateral* knee replacement, the sequence of events is nearly the same and includes:

- Suture removal at 2–3 weeks (3 weeks in patients of rheumatoid arthritis) **(Fig. 1)**
- Walker aided ambulation for 1–2 weeks → walking stick/ cane for another 2–3 weeks → independent ambulation (by 4–6 weeks)
- Stair climbing at 3–4 weeks
- Car driving at 3 months

The following features need to be assessed at every follow-up visit after surgery:

- Local skin, wound, and soft tissue condition
- Clinical assessment for range of movement and function (KSS scoring, pain, and function)
- Pain scoring using visual analogue scale (VAS) as well as pain component of KSS
- Radiological assessment (including radiological KSS score) **(Fig. 2)**.

Chapter 21

Thromboprophylaxis Update

In the early postoperative period, deep venous thrombosis (DVT) is a major known complication and life-threatening if it embolizes to the lung, pulmonary embolism (PE). Asymptomatic DVT has been reported in up to 50–70% of patients who undergo total knee arthroplasty (TKA).

Figure 1 shows the cascade of thrombus generation and the possible intervention points, which have sparked research into and advocated many direct oral anticoagulants (DOACs). Postoperative ultrasonography or venography can reveal the presence of thrombi quite successfully. Prevention must be routinely provided with multiple modalities, which include early mobilization, the use of compression stockings, passive and assisted ankle/foot pumps, and chemoprophylaxis **(Figs. 2 and 3)**. Prophylaxis with anticoagulant

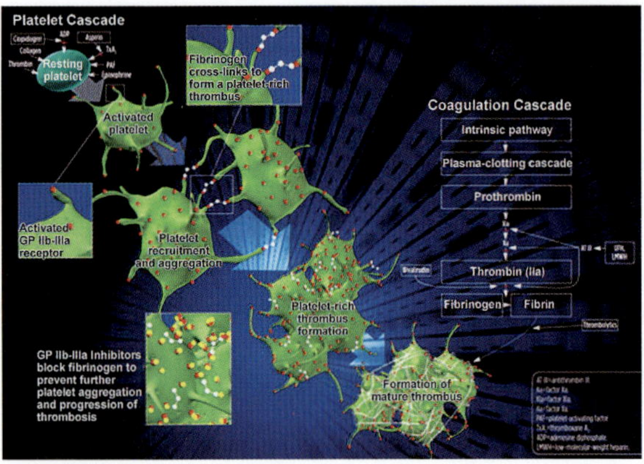

FIG. 1: The cascade of thrombus generation and points of intervention in prevention of deep venous thrombosis (DVT).

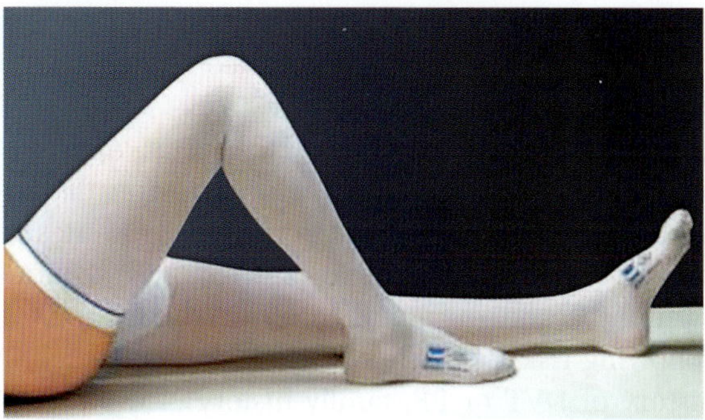

FIG. 2: Graduated compression stockings used as mechanical deep venous thrombosis (DVT) prophylaxis.

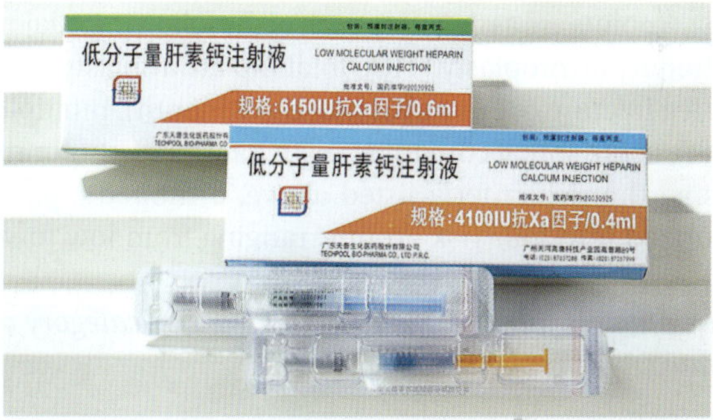

FIG. 3: Low-molecular-weight heparin (LMWH) used in deep venous thrombosis (DVT) chemoprophylaxis.

medications, as well as the adjunctive use of mechanical devices, is essential.

The most effective treatment protocol for a patient must be determined on a case-by-case basis and account for the risk-benefit ratio in each situation. A risk stratification protocol (developed by the ACCP) is recommended to determine the appropriate level and method of treatment. Risk factors for DVT (and PE) are grouped according to severity and are added to produce an overall risk factor score, which corresponds to a low through a very high potential for DVT development.

In risk factor assessment, 1 point is assigned to each of the following: Age (41–60 years), minor surgery, history of major surgery within 1 month, pregnancy or postpartum within 1 month, varicose veins, inflammatory bowel disease, swelling of legs, obesity [body mass index (BMI) >25 kg/m^2], and oral contraceptives, patch, or hormone replacement therapy.

Each of the following is assigned 2 points: Age (>60 years), malignancy or current chemotherapy or radiation therapy, major surgery (>45 minutes), laparoscopic surgery (>45 minutes), confined to bed (>72 hours), immobilizing cast (<1 month), central venous access (<1 month), and tourniquet time (>45 minutes).

The following risk factors are assigned 3 points each: Age (>75 years), history of DVT or PE, family history of thrombosis, factor V Leiden/activated protein C resistance, medical patient with risk factors (myocardial infarction, congestive heart failure, or chronic obstructive pulmonary disease), congenital, or acquired thrombophilia.

Finally, 5 points are assigned to each of the following: Major elective lower-extremity arthroplasty [TKA/total hip arthroplasty (THA)], hip, pelvis, or leg fracture (<1 month), stroke (<1 month), multiple trauma (<1 month), acute spinal cord injury with paralysis (<1 month).

By using the risk criteria listed above, orthopedic patients can be categorized into four risk groups, ranging from low to very high **(Table 1)**.

All our patients fall in the very high DVT risk category and need appropriate DVT prophylaxis.

EUROPEAN RECOMMENDATIONS

The updated European guidelines on perioperative prophylaxis of venous thromboembolism (VTE) in patients undergoing inpatient orthopedic surgery (August 2024) included many recommendations. We have listed the guidelines for TKA/THA surgery as under:

- For evaluation of VTE and bleeding risk, routine patient-specific preoperative evaluation, based on procedure type and planned postoperative course (fast-track or standard), is suggested.

Table 1: The risk levels and overall deep venous thrombosis (DVT) incidence based on risk factor scores.

Risk factor score	0–1	2	3–4	5+
DVT incidence	2%	10–20%	20–40%	40–80%
Risk level	Low	Moderate	High	Very high

- After THA, TKA, or hip fracture surgery (HFS), pharmacologic VTE prophylaxis is recommended over no prophylaxis.
- For patients undergoing high-VTE-risk procedures (TKA/THA) who have a high risk of bleeding, mechanical VTE prophylaxis is suggested in preference to pharmacologic prophylaxis.
- For patients undergoing high-VTE-risk procedures (TKA/THA) who have no high risk of bleeding, pharmacologic VTE prophylaxis with LMWH or DOAC is suggested in preference to no prophylaxis; no recommendation can be made either for or against aspirin.
- After fast-track THA or TKA, pharmacologic VTE prophylaxis with LMWH, DOAC, or aspirin is recommended over no prophylaxis.
- After fast-track THA, TKA, or HFS, pharmacologic VTE prophylaxis with LMWH or DOAC is recommended over no prophylaxis; prophylaxis with aspirin is recommended over no prophylaxis; prophylaxis with LMWH or DOAC is recommended over no prophylaxis.

EUROPEAN SOCIETY OF ANAESTHESIOLOGY

European Society of Anaesthesiology (ESA) issued the following guidelines regarding prophylaxis for VTE in elderly patients undergoing surgery (September 2017):

- The risk for postoperative VTE is increased in patients >70 years and those presenting with comorbidities (cardiovascular disorders, malignancy, or renal insufficiency); therefore, risk stratification, correction of modifiable risks, and sustained perioperative thromboprophylaxis are essential in this patient population.
- In elderly, careful prescription of postoperative VTE prophylaxis and early postoperative mobilization is recommended. *Recommend multifaceted interventions for VTE prophylaxis in elderly and frail patients, including pneumatic compression devices, LMWH, and/or DOACs after knee or hip replacement.*
- Early mobilization and use of nonpharmacologic means of thromboprophylaxis should be exploited.
- Timing and dosing of chemoprophylaxis may be adopted from the younger population. DOACs are effective and well tolerated in the elderly; statins may not replace pharmacologic thromboprophylaxis.

- In elderly patients, identification of comorbidities increasing the risk for VTE (e.g., congestive heart failure, pulmonary circulation disorder, renal failure, lymphoma, metastatic cancer, obesity, arthritis, postmenopausal estrogen therapy, anemia, and coagulopathy) and correction where possible.
- In elderly with renal failure, low-dose unfractionated heparin (UFH) may be used (or weight-adjusted dosing of LMWH).

ACCP RECOMMENDATIONS

The 10th edition of the ACCP guidelines for patients undergoing major orthopedic surgery (THA, TKA, or HFS) included the following (August 2016):

- In patients undergoing TKA or THA, *LMWH, fondaparinux, apixaban, dabigatran, rivaroxaban, low-dose unfractionated heparin (LDUH), adjusted-dose vitamin K antagonist (VKA), aspirin, or an intermittent pneumatic compression (IPC) device for at least 10–14 days is preferable to no prophylaxis.*
- In patients who receive LMWH, prophylaxis should be started at least 12 hours preoperatively or postoperatively.
- Regardless of concomitant IPC device use or duration of treatment, LMWH is favored over alternative recommended agents. During the hospital stay, dual prophylaxis with an IPC device and an antithrombotic agent is suggested.
- In patients who are at increased risk for bleeding, an IPC device or no prophylaxis is favored over pharmacologic prophylaxis.
- *Thromboprophylaxis should be extended in the outpatient period for up to 35 days from the day of surgery.*
- In patients who refuse or will not cooperate with injections or an IPC device, apixaban or dabigatran (or, if these are unavailable, rivaroxaban or adjusted-dose VKA) is recommended.

NOT RECOMMENDED

- In patients who are at increased risk for bleeding or in whom both mechanical and pharmacologic prophylaxis are contraindicated, placement of an inferior vena cava filter is not recommended.
- In patients who are asymptomatic after surgery, Doppler ultrasound screening before discharge is not recommended.

ANESTHESIA IN PATIENTS RECEIVING THROMBOPROPHYLAXIS

Anticoagulant prophylaxis should be used with caution in patients receiving spinal or indwelling catheter epidural anesthesia. Although the risk of spinal hematoma is very small (0.0025% with spinal anesthesia and 0.03% with epidural anesthesia), care should be taken to delay the initiation of thromboprophylaxis for at least 2 hours after catheter removal. Patients with known bleeding disorders should not receive preoperative prophylaxis if they are to receive spinal anesthesia.

In cases of traumatic spinal tap with bloody spinal fluid, postoperative administration of thromboprophylaxis should be done with caution.

INITIATION OF THROMBOPROPHYLAXIS

In Europe, it is common practice to begin anticoagulant prophylaxis 10–12 hours before surgery. In North America, the practice is to begin treatment 12–24 hours following surgery. Meta-analyses suggest little advantage for preoperative initiation. Patients with a high risk of bleeding should have the first postoperative dose delayed 12–24 hours after surgery.

OUR PROTOCOL

Low-molecular-weight heparin is our drug of choice for inpatient chemoprophylaxis. Daily subcutaneous LMW heparin (enoxaparin) is initiated starting from the evening of surgery, till 12 hours after removal of catheter, or till discharge. Thereafter we recommend oral anticoagulants for 4 weeks. NOACs (such as apixaban 2.5 mg twice a day) are now used routinely by us in chemoprophylaxis of DVT following TKA/THA. Patients with a high risk of bleeding are given mechanical prophylaxis alone.

INFERIOR VENA CAVA FILTERS

Patients felt to be at particularly high risk for VTE development and who have a clinical contraindication to prophylactic anticoagulation are the most likely to have an inferior vena cava filter (IVCF) placed.

Inferior vena cava filter placement in the combat theater may be used for:

- Primary prophylaxis (no evidence of VTE disease at the time of placement)
- Secondary prophylaxis (documented DVT) of PE in the TKA/THA/polytrauma patient

The vast majority of IVCF devices placed in the combat theater are retrievable inferior vena cava filters (RIVCFs). RIVCFs are preferred to avoid some of the long-term complications of filter placement.

If a DVT or PE is identified, then therapeutic anticoagulation is necessary per current guidelines, and if it is contraindicated, then an IVCF should be considered.

Chapter 22

Complications

Total knee arthroplasty (TKA) surgery is fraught with complications. These are however identifiable, correctible, treatable, sometimes completely reversible, and *usually preventable.*

Early complications can occur intraoperatively, perioperatively, and postoperatively and may be:

- Those specific to the operation
- Due to general complications of the anesthetic
- Associated medical/surgical complications (coexistent medical comorbidities)

Operative complications include blood loss, neurovascular injury, intraoperative fractures, early setting of cement, as well as anesthetic problems (hypotension, arrhythmia, giddiness, vomiting, etc.).

Perioperative complications include blood loss, infection, early hemorrhage and wound breakdown, intra- and postoperative fractures, and medical complications (cardiovascular, respiratory, renal, electrolyte, and other medical problems).

In the early postoperative period, deep venous thrombosis (DVT) and pulmonary embolism (PE) are major dangers. Prevention is routinely provided with early mobilization, thrombo-embolus deterrent (TED) stockings, foot pumps, and anticoagulant chemoprophylaxis, and the prevention is covered in the chapter of thromboprophylaxis. Once developed, thrombolytic therapy is recommended (systemic preferred over catheter-directed) in hypotensive individuals with an acute PE. Those with high-risk PE presenting in shock should undergo systemic thrombolysis; when thrombolysis is contraindicated owing to a high risk of bleeding, consider surgical thrombectomy or catheter-directed thrombolysis.

Acute DVT may be treated in an outpatient setting with low-molecular-weight heparin (LMWH). Patients with low-risk PE may be safely discharged early from hospital or receive only outpatient treatment with LMWH, followed by vitamin K anticoagulants (VKA), although non-vitamin K-dependent oral anticoagulants may be as effective but safer than the LMWH/VKA regimen. Anticoagulant therapy is recommended for 3–12 months depending on the site of thrombosis and on the ongoing presence of risk factors. If DVT recurs, if a chronic hypercoagulability is identified, or if the PE is life threatening, lifetime anticoagulation therapy may be recommended. This treatment protocol has a cumulative risk of bleeding complication of less than 12%.

Infection is rare (<1% of cases) following TKA. Prophylactic antibiotics (second-generation cephalosporin and aminoglycosides) are used routinely for the first 48–72 hours. When diagnosed in the early perioperative period, it is treated urgently with the debridement, antibiotics, and implant retention (DAIR) procedure (debridement and implant retention), followed by 6 weeks of antibiotics (as per culture reports). Usually, the tibial insert is exchanged at this time to prevent reseeding of infection from potential spaces.

Neurovascular complications are rare. The lateral popliteal nerve may be injured in severe valgus deformity. Tourniquet paralysis may also occur as a rare problem. Major vessel injury may occur in revision procedures or in the rare case in which anatomy is abnormal. Fine attention to operating technique and surgical principles, with adroit handling of tissues and efficient teamwork, reduces operating time to a minimum and thus avoid exposing the wound unnecessarily or for an inordinate amount of time.

Late problems associated with TKA are late infection, insert wear, mid-flexion instability, and aseptic loosening. Periprosthetic fracture, dislocation, patellar malalignment issues, and arthrofibrosis are other problems that occur but less commonly **(Fig. 1)**.

Improved instrumentation and computer-aided surgery have reduced malalignment and incorrect insertions, thereby minimizing malalignment issues (varus/valgus and patellar tracking).

It is important to keep the subsequent revision procedure in mind while planning and executing a primary total knee replacement. Cortical bone including the medullary cavity must be preserved as much as possible (stemless prosthesis), and soft tissue preservation (especially ligaments) is equally important.

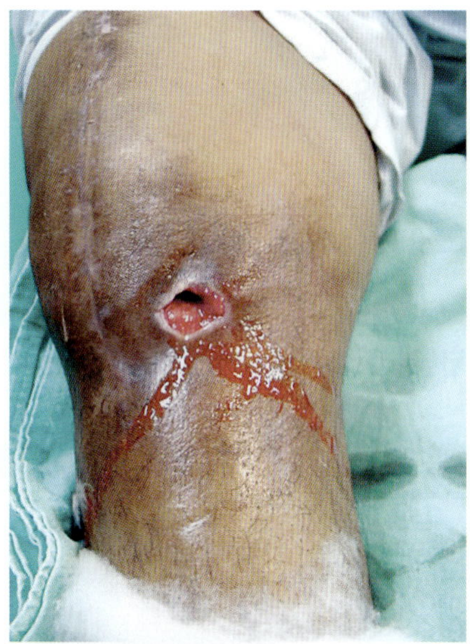

FIG. 1: Clinical picture of infection following total knee arthroplasty (TKA) surgery (late complication).

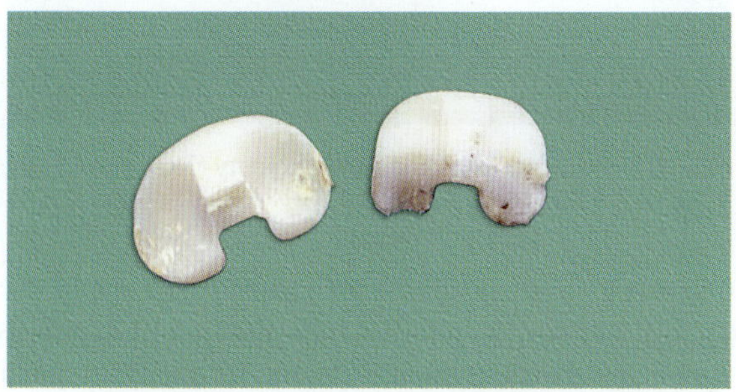

FIG. 2: Wear in retrieved polyethylene insert.

Wear is less of a problem in the knee than the hip. The coefficient of friction between polyethylene and cobalt-chromium alloy (commonly used for femoral components) has been reported to be 0.03–0.16, with excellent wear rates. Highly cross-linked poly is now available, and with newer cobalt-chrome tibial trays, the wear rates are drastically reduced. Mobile bearings have significantly reduced surface stresses, but an increased risk of subluxation **(Figs. 2 and 3)**.

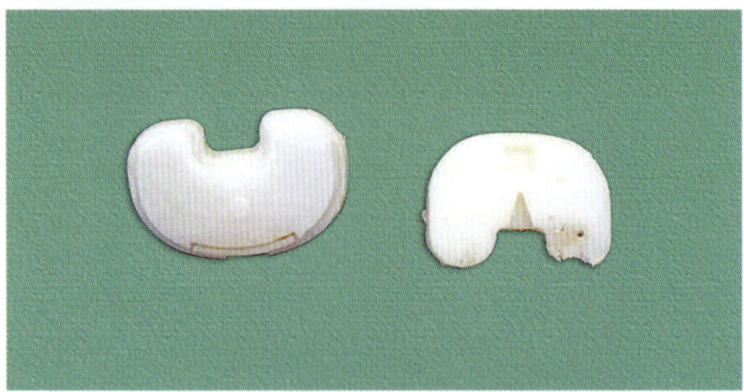

FIG. 3: Backside wear on tibial component.

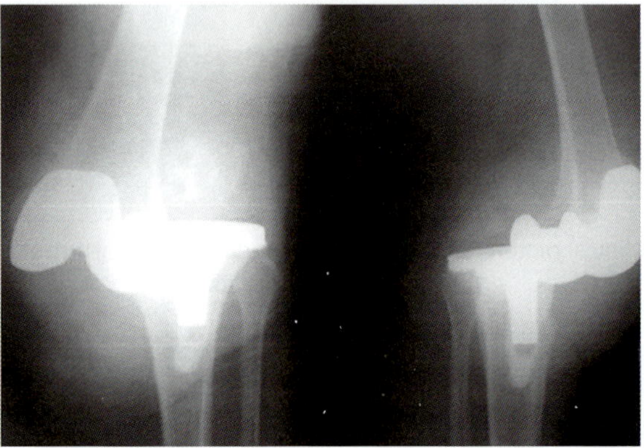

FIG. 4: Dislocated total knee arthroplasty (TKA) prosthesis.

Osteolysis is a major problem with polyethylene and metal wear fragments. The pathology consists of a significant synovitis caused by wear particles in the synovial cavity. These wear particles are forced along the lines of least resistance, and the inflamed synovium tracks down the vascular bony foramina around the joint. Severe osteolysis can also occur in pigmented villonodular synovitis and in patients with hemophilia. Preoperative assessment and knowledge of previous injuries and operations are important.

Dislocation of a TKA prosthesis demonstrates poor soft tissue balancing. Inadequate spacer insertion, poor ligament balancing, excessive bone resection, and/or malrotation of the prosthesis can cause this unusual complication **(Fig. 4)**.

Complications associated with the patellar component include patella tendon avulsion [often associated with a previous high tibial

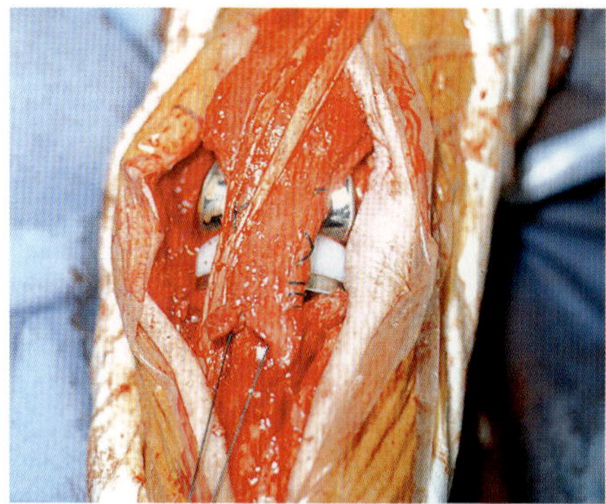
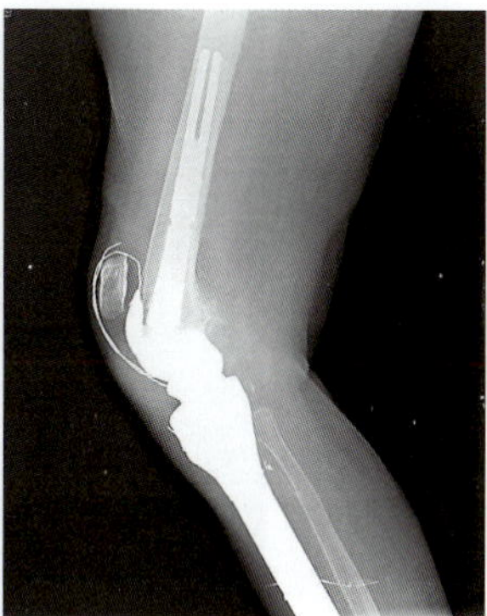

FIG. 5: Patellar tendon avulsion during revision total knee replacement (TKR) stabilized with modified detensioning stitch.

osteotomy (HTO)] **(Fig. 5)**, patellofemoral instability (inadequate soft tissue balancing), and component failure due to recurrent instability, loosening, or fracture. Patella clunk has also been seen with posterior cruciate-sacrificing prosthesis designs.

Fixation of components with or without cement is still debated widely. Studies comparing both methods have revealed little, if any, differences. Bioactive coatings such as hydroxyapatite have been used to enhance uncemented fixation, with favorable medium- to long-term results. Prosthetic loosening is the most common cause of long-term failure in TKA, due to osteolysis from wear-particle synovitis.

The differential diagnosis in the early perioperative period is between superficial and deep infection. Blood tests [erythrocyte sedimentation rate (ESR) and C-reactive protein (CRP)] are not helpful. Elevated temperature is an indication, and the presence of a red, inflamed joint confirms the diagnosis. Saving the prosthesis is possible if early exploration and thorough synovectomy are performed. In late infections, complete removal of the prostheses is indicated, with removal of all components and cement. A two-stage revision, excision of all infected tissue (complete synovectomy and thorough washout), and prolonged antibiotics are the norm **(Fig. 6)**.

Differential diagnosis of chronic pain in the late stage includes aseptic loosening, arthrofibrosis, sympathetic dystrophy, and, possibly, referred pain from the hip or spine. Arthrolysis may benefit severe arthrofibrosis.

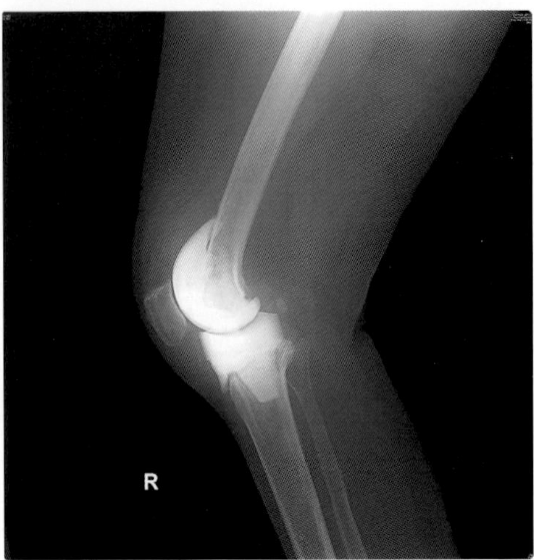

FIG. 6: X-ray of knee following first-stage revision (with antibiotic-loaded cement spacer).

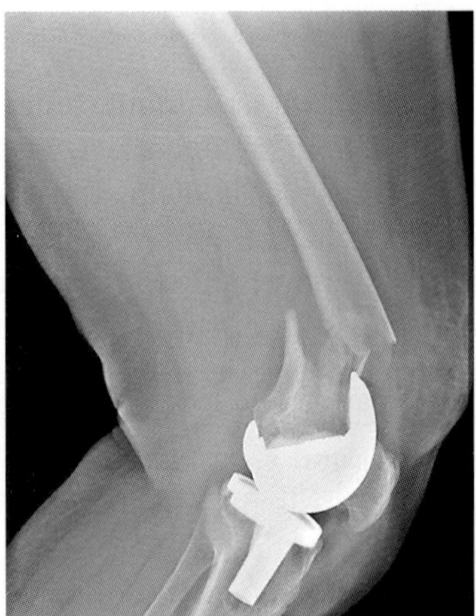

FIG. 7: Supracondylar periprosthetic femoral fracture.

Periprosthetic fracture is a rare complication (1–5%) and is usually the result of trauma. Therefore, it is treated on an individual basis, depending on the site and type of fracture. Other causes include notching of the femoral component and osteoporosis. It may be necessary in some cases to insert a large-stem prosthesis. Femoral fracture is the most common type of fracture and usually occurs in the supracondylar region **(Fig. 7)**.

Chapter 23

Issues

POSTERIOR CRUCIATE LIGAMENT (TABLE 1)

Table 1: Criteria of posterior cruciate ligament (PCL) sacrificing and retaining.

Criteria	*PCL-sacrificing*	*PCL-retaining*
Bone cuts	More as notch is cut	Less
Posterior femoral rollback	Effective → less wear	Less effective → more wear (if PCL is tight)
Range of motion (ROM)	Potentially less (varying reports)	Potentially more (varying reports)
Wear	? Less	? More
Proprioception and balance	Absent → difficulty in stair climbing	Present → better stair climbing
Patellofemoral joint function	Possible "patellar clunk syndrome" (older models)	Better
Loosening	Increased stress on cement-bone interface (if concurrent instability)	Resistance to translation

Author's Preferred Method of Treatment

The author always sacrifices the posterior cruciate ligament (PCL), the technique is simpler, and there is no conclusive proof that PCL-retention produces better results **(Figs. 1A and B)**.

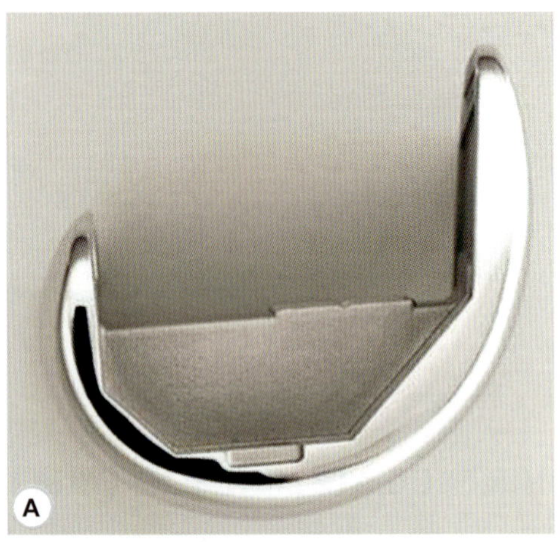

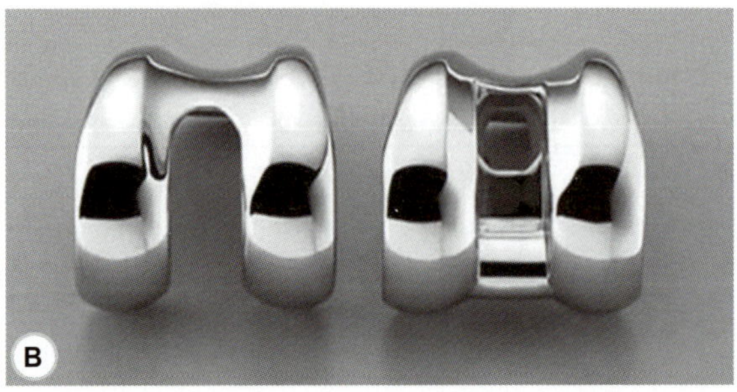

FIGS. 1A AND B: (A) PCL-substituting femoral prosthesis. (B) PCL-retaining versus PCL-substituting femoral prosthesis.

(PCL: posterior cruciate ligament)

PATELLA (TABLE 2)

Table 2: Criteria of patellar resurfacing and nonresurfacing.

Criteria	*Patellar resurfacing*	*Patellar nonresurfacing*
Postoperative anterior knee pain	Absent	May be present
Stair climbing	Improved (better quadriceps strength)	Less (lower quadriceps strength)
Functional scores	Better	Lower
Complications	Possible (fractures, loosening)	No such case

Author's Preferred Method of Treatment

We now routinely replace the patella (patella replacement). Shaving off the eroded cartilage and removal of osteophytes is performed routinely. We recommend patellaplasty only in young patients with preserved cartilage **(Figs. 2A and B)**.

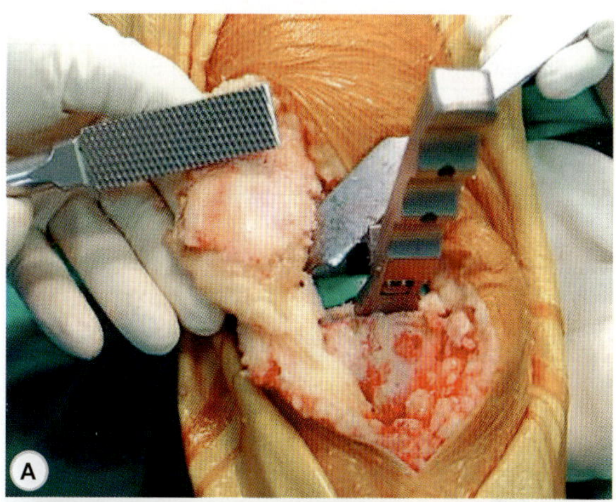

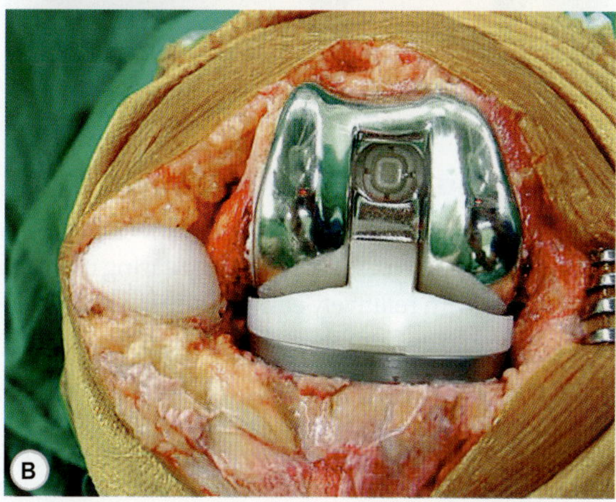

FIGS. 2A AND B: (A) Intraoperative photograph of patellaplasty; and (B) Patellar prosthesis.

BEARING TYPE (TABLE 3)

Table 3: Criteria of fixed bearing and mobile bearing.

Criteria	*Fixed bearing*	*Mobile bearing*
Biomechanics	Compromised	Better (permits rotational stress)
Wear	More	Less
Range of motion (ROM)	Lower	Better
Rotation	Design does not permit	Design permits rotational stress

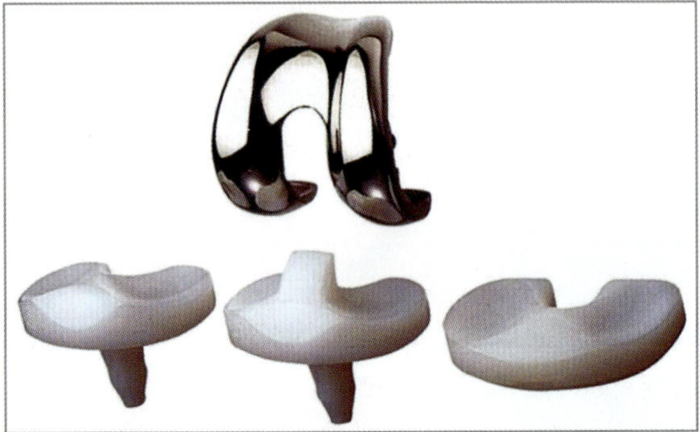

FIG. 3: Fixed and mobile-bearing tibial inserts.

Author's Preferred Method of Treatment

Fixed bearing implants are the gold standard especially in elderly with unstable joints. We reserve use of the mobile-bearing meniscus design for younger patients with relatively early arthritis, with physiologically undamaged and stable collateral ligaments **(Fig. 3)**.

CEMENT (TABLE 4)

Table 4: Criteria of uncemented and cemented.

Criteria	*Uncemented*	*Cemented*
Fixation strength	Initially lower, then high	High, then gradually lessens
Bone preservation and revision	Better and easier	Like cemented hips bone loss is extensive during revision

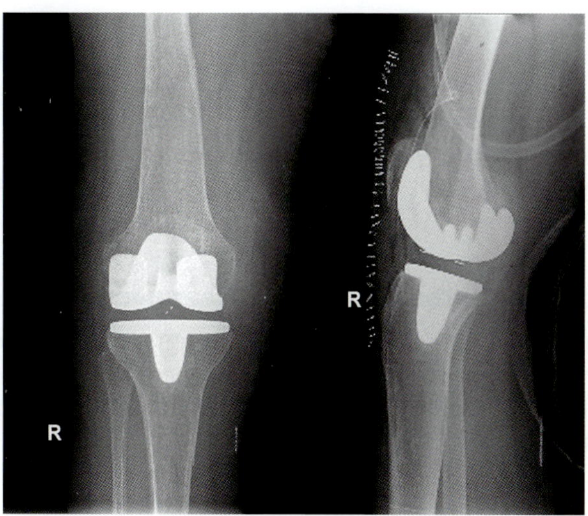

FIG. 4: Uncemented total knee arthroplasty (TKA)—anteroposterior (AP) and lateral views (TiNi knee).

Author's Preferred Method of Treatment

We have very limited experience with cementless knee systems. However, the future holds more in store with development of improved fixation modalities (namely, surface coating with metal particles/hydroxyapatite). We have limited experience with hydroxyapatite-coated knee implants. We have a reason to believe that cementless systems may be more commonly used in the near future **(Fig. 4)**.

USE OF TOURNIQUETS AND DRAINS

- Although, there are proponents of tourniquet (better cement integration, less bleeding during surgery, and reduced anesthesia/blood requirements due to reduced surgical time), many surgeons have adopted the *no tourniquet or use only during cementation* approach, citing benefits of less postoperative thigh pain, reduced incidence of deep vein thrombosis (DVT), and reduced muscle weakness. A middle path is to apply the tourniquet before surgery, inflate it during cementation to improve cement interdigitation, and deflate it at the end of cementing, to ensure ligation, and cauterization of bleeders before closure.
- Although drains were used extensively in the past, most surgeons today avoid the use of drains to reduce risk of an additional

foreign body (communicating with the external environment) and therefore infection, and the possible complication of partial/inability to remove the drains due to suture material enclosing the drains. However, in patients who have been on antiplatelet/anticoagulant medication before surgery, it is a good idea to keep a no-suction drain for the first 24 hours to prevent hematoma formation, and subsequent risk infection.

Author's Preferred Method of Treatment

We routinely use tourniquets for the procedure as we tend to finish the surgery within an hour and have stopped using drains unless indicated in patients having bleeding tendencies/antiplatelet medication.

Chapter 24

Current Day Economics of Total Knee Arthroplasty

Cost can prove to be a constraint for widespread acceptance of this hugely successful and beneficial surgical procedure, even though the implant costs have been brought under the purview of the Indian Government regulation. Estimated implant cost is ₹80,000 (range, ₹75,000–105,000).

Apart from the implant, major factors affecting the cost include the use of modern operating rooms which utilize many of the following:

- Laminar air flow systems, body exhaust systems
- Cement vacuum mixers, centrifuge, and antibiotic-loaded cement packets
- Pulsatile lavage systems **(Fig. 1)**
- Disposable gowns and drapes
- High-end perioperative antibiotics
- Chemo and physical thromboprophylaxis systems

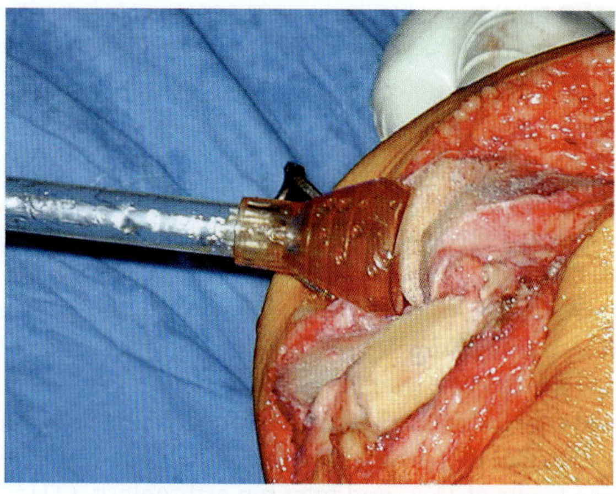

FIG. 1: Pulsatile lavage system.

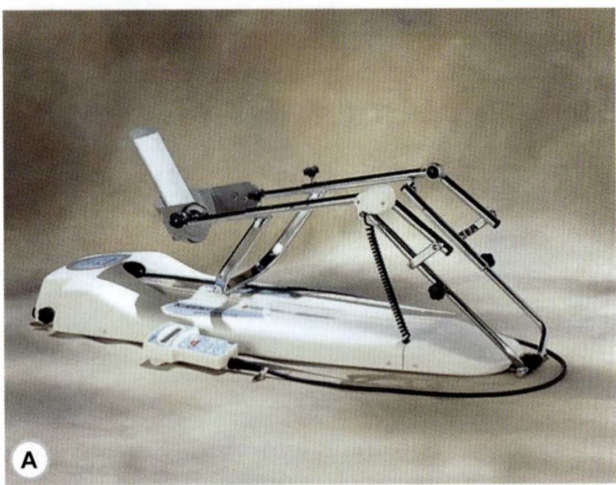

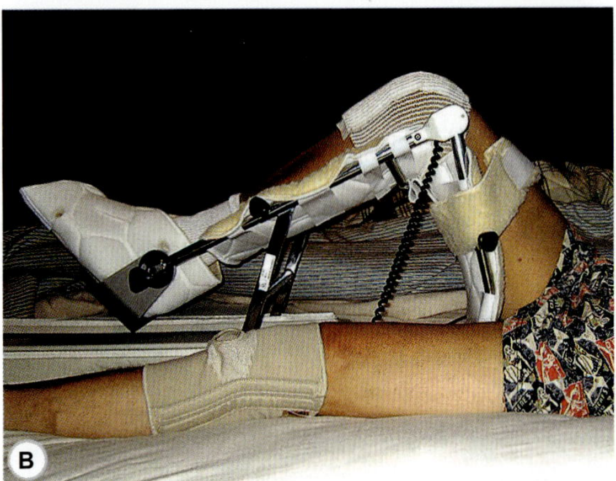

FIGS. 2A AND B: (A) Basic CPM machine. (B) ROM is achieved early using the CPM machine (specially in fusion take down TKA surgeries).

(CPM: continuous passive motion; ROM: range of motion; TKA: total knee arthroplasty)

- Blood and blood products
- Physiotherapy modalities [including continuous passive motion (CPM) machine] **(Figs. 2A and B)**

The overall surgery cost of a unilateral total knee arthroplasty (TKA) in a public hospital in India (as of September 2024) is approximately ₹85,000 (range, ₹75,000–100,000), while the same surgery will cost the average patient approximately ₹250,000 (range, ₹175,000–350,000) in a private hospital. While one would like to cut costs, some facets of TKA [and total hip arthroplasty (THA)] cannot be compromised on, and these include infection, implant durability, and thromboprophylaxis.

INFECTION

Bacteria need dust particles to be suspended in air, macroparticles (>10 μm) are likely to settle within 1 hour and are clinically important, whereas microparticles (<1 μm) remain suspended for long durations.

- *Air filters* that are designed to filter particles <1 μm are ideal but may not be cost effective. Ultra-clean filters (laminar air flow systems) change air in the operation theater (OT) nearly 400–600 times every hour but are expensive (cost >₹15 lakhs) **(Figs. 3A and B)**. If OTs are used only for clean orthopedic procedures,

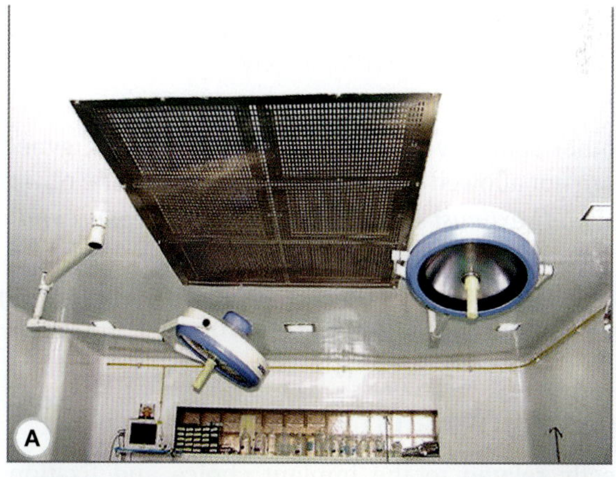

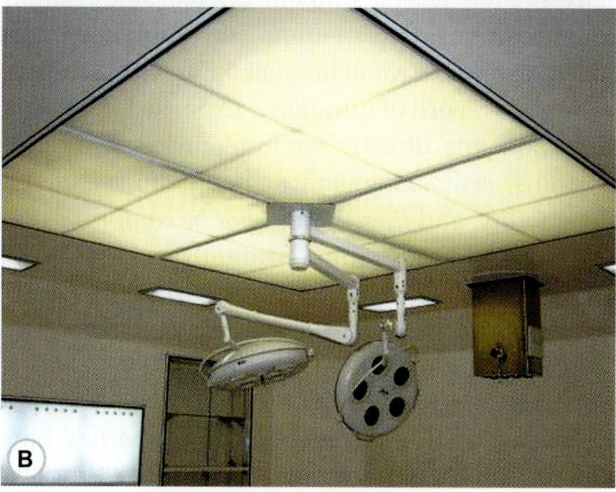

FIGS. 3A AND B: Laminar air flow systems used in operation theaters.

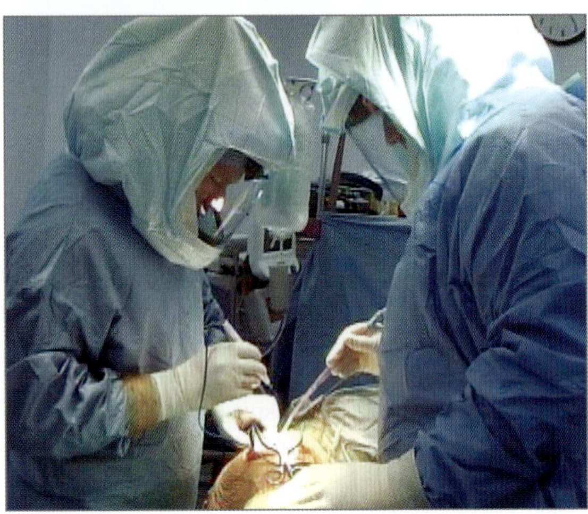

FIG. 4: Body exhaust systems being used during total knee arthroplasty (TKA) surgery.

and other specialty surgeons (general surgeons, gynecologists, etc.) are not allowed the same OT, this cost can be obviated.

- Use of *body exhaust systems* and *disposable gowns and drapes* is not essential **(Fig. 4)**.
- *Antibiotics* are essential (ideally recommended for prophylaxis for 24–48 hours and cannot be compromised on).

IMPLANT DURABILITY

It is directly related to the implant choice and fixation to host bone through cement. Use of unproven implant systems is not recommended, as these have neither all the essential instrumentation nor a proven track record of durability. Expense for implants is one-time, and responsible directly for implant longevity. Sometimes, revision systems, extensions, and augmentations may be needed for implant stability, and *these should not be compromised on at all.* It is also essential to keep trauma fixation sets ready and available to handle any possible eventuality at the earliest instead of waiting for the system to be made available with consequent delay and prolonged wound exposure.

- *Vacuum mixers* reduce cement porosity and void generation, thereby improving strength and fixation properties, but are more essential in THR for femoral stem fixation, and this cost may be

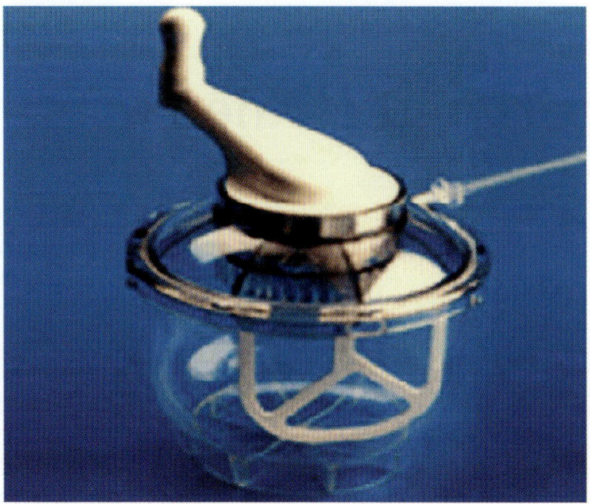

FIG. 5: Basic vacuum mixing device.

avoided in total knee replacement (TKR) by appropriate manual cement mixing technique (gentle mixing, allowing for bubbles to escape, initial mixing till semiliquid state, and then allowing self-setting, preventing blood-cement mixing, etc.) **(Fig. 5)**.

- *Antibiotic-loaded cement* is more expensive, and its use may be reserved for special conditions (prior infection, revision TKA surgery, immunocompromised conditions such as rheumatoid arthritis (RA), diabetes mellitus (DM), postorgan transplant, and for patient on disease-modifying antirheumatic drugs (DMRDs)/steroids, etc.), minimizing costs.
- *Blood* interferes with cement properties as well as cement fixation and needs to be carefully removed during the cementing process.
- And here, the role of *tourniquets* and *pulsatile lavage systems* is invaluable. Disposable pulsavacs generally cost ₹3,000 (range, 2,800–4,000), and should not be compromised on.

THROMBOPROPHYLAXIS

The role of thromboprophylaxis has been stressed in adequate detail in the previous chapters, and therefore we strongly adequate the routine use of long-term (3–4 weeks) of oral agents after discharge following TKA.

Chapter 25

Compartmental Knee Arthroplasty

Not all knee arthritic patients need a total knee arthroplasty (TKA). When only a single compartment is involved in the arthritic process (isolated medial or lateral compartment, or the patellofemoral compartment), unicompartment arthroplasty is possible. Occasionally, when two of the three knee compartments are affected, dual (or bicompartment arthroplasty) replacement is possible today.

UNICOMPARTMENT KNEE ARTHROPLASTY

Since the discovery of Ahlback in 1968 that 85% of knees with clinical osteoarthritis (OA) have isolated medial compartment degeneration, unicompartment knee arthroplasty (UKA) has been an effective and minimally invasive alternative to total knee arthroplasty (TKA). In a typical Indian arthroplasty practice, <10% of patients with OA have isolated medial compartment involvement and about 1% have isolated lateral compartmental involvement.

Optimal treatment of unicompartmental arthritis remains controversial. Nonoperative treatment activity modification, non-steroidal anti-inflammatory drugs (NSAIDs), chondroprotective agents, intra-articular injections, orthotic devices is recommended for mild cases. Surgical options are also many, and include osteochondral autograft, autologous chondrocyte implantation, osteoarticular allograft, arthroscopic joint debridement/microfractures, distal femoral/proximal tibial osteotomy, unicondylar knee replacement, and total knee replacement [and more recently the unicompartmental interpositional implant (ConforMIS iForma)].

Evolution of Implants

The McKeever and MacIntosh UKA prosthesis was first developed in the late 1950s to address the problem of unicompartment arthritis, with uniformly poor results. Since then, better implant designs, proper and precise instrumentation, experience in surgical techniques, and evolution of MIS techniques has resulted in the reemergence of UKA. Goodfellow and Connor (1980s) introduced the Oxford knee which heralded a new era in UKA and has been the biggest advancement in the field of partial knee arthroplasty.

Types of Unicompartment Knee Arthroplasty Implants

The UKA systems are classified according to bone cut preparations (resurfacing vs. inset) and bearing surfaces (all poly vs. modular metal-backed) (fixed-bearing vs. mobile-bearing) **(Figs. 1A and B)**.

In resurfacing systems (viz. Marmor, St. George, and Repicci), implants are placed on to the subchondral bone after minimal bone resection. Limited guiding jigs make resurfacing techniques surgically challenging. In contrast, the inset technique (Porous Coated Anatomic knee and Miller-Galante) relies on proper angular bone cuts as in TKA **(Fig. 1A)**.

Bearing surfaces may be all poly or modular, and fixed or mobile. Fixed-bearing metal-backed UKA is technically straightforward with relatively simple instrumentation and has consistently shown good mid-term and long-term survivorship. Fixed-bearing designs

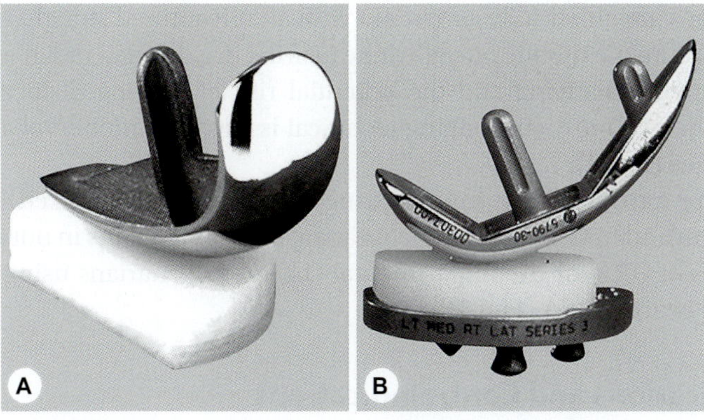

FIGS. 1A AND B: (A) Repicci unicompartmental knee prosthesis with all-polyethylene tibial component. (B) Metal-backed tibial component.

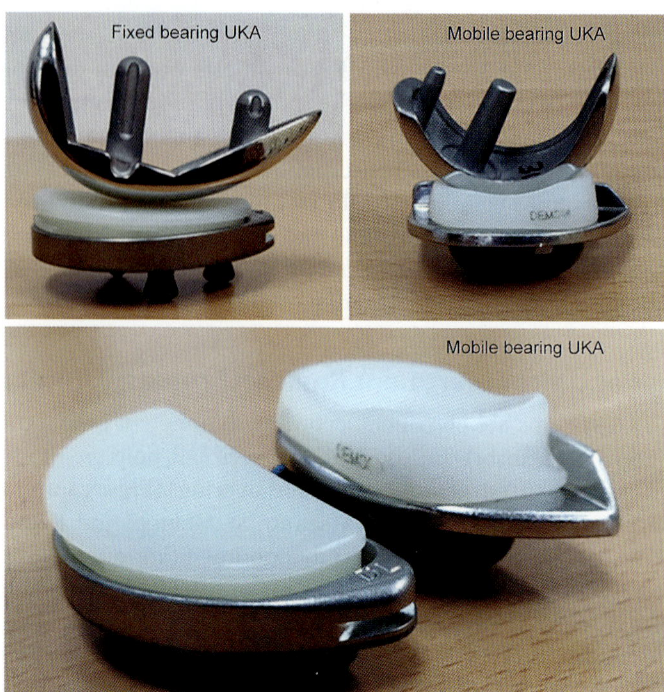

FIG. 2: Fixed-bearing UKA and mobile-bearing UKA designs.

(UKA: unicompartment knee arthroplasty)

have round-on-flat or slightly dished geometries. Mobile-bearing designs are either fully congruent with an uncaptured straight track or capture the mobile polyethylene bearing in a dovetail radial track. Ligament balancing and the potential risk of bearing dislocation are the two most challenging technical issues with mobile-bearing designs **(Fig. 2)**.

We have used the fixed bearing monobloc metal-backed UKA system and have observed encouraging mid-term results in our case series of UKA for tricompartmental OA in octogenarians using this fixed bearing UKA **(Fig. 3)**.

Indications and Contraindications

The UKA is either done for middle-aged females as their "first arthroplasty" or for elderly individuals as their "last arthroplasty".

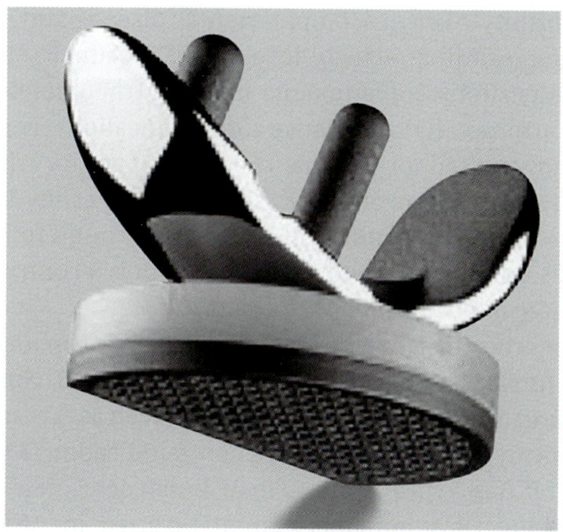

FIG. 3: Allegretto unicompartment knee system (Zimmer).

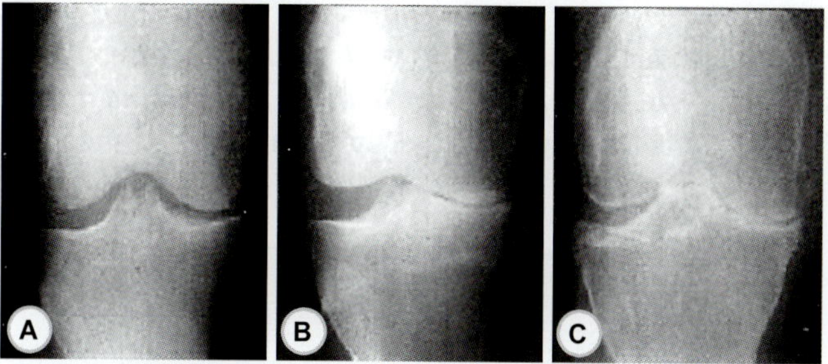

FIGS. 4A TO C: Ahlback osteoarthritis (OA) stages II, III, and IV.

According to Kozinn and Scott, the ideal patient must be >60 years old, weigh <180 lbs (82 kg), must have low activity levels, with minimal rest pain. Better results occur in the presence of a minimum range of motion (ROM) arc of 90°, with no >5° flexion contracture, and a correctable maximal anatomical coronal deformity of 10° varus/15° valgus. Radiological indications for UKA are 50% unicompartment joint space collapse (Ahlback II and III) and complete collapse (Ahlback III and IV) on standing X-ray views **(Figs. 4A to C)**.

Contraindications are more clearly defined. Symptomatic patellofemoral disease, cruciate and collateral ligament instability, obesity, decreased ROM (loss of extension>15°, flexion<90°, and varus/

valgus deformity >10°), tricompartmental disease and unrealistic expectations regarding activity levels, and prosthetic survival are all contraindications. Inflammatory diseases (rheumatoid arthritis, crystalloid arthropathy) are relative contraindications. Traditionally, UKA was not advised for patients <60 years of age, or with obesity, but recently a few surgeons have shown good results in younger patients too. Body mass index (BMI) has been found to be a better indicator, as a small bony body in a large man is a contraindication but not a large bony body in a large man.

Anterior cruciate ligament (ACL) insufficiency can increase poly wear and implant loosening in some designs and consequently higher failure rates. Mediolateral instability (seen as "kissing lesions" intraoperatively) is also considered a contraindication **(Fig. 5)**.

Lateral UKA is *contraindicated* in ACL-deficient knees. Similarly, mobile-bearing UKA implants cannot be used in ACL-deficient knee because of the propensity for meniscal dislocation. UKA can judiciously be done in older patients without a functional ACL but with no symptoms of instability.

The final decision of whether to proceed with a UKA or TKA in a patient with doubtful ligaments and other compartment arthritis should be taken intraoperatively; with an open mind to convert to TKA if indicated (significant arthritis in other compartments,

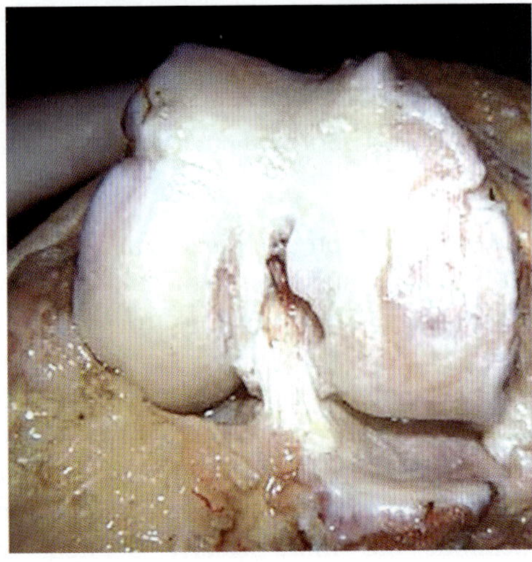

FIG. 5: "Kissing lesion" on lateral femoral condyle (medial wall) indicates medial lateral instability.

absent or nonfunctional ACL, or when the surgeon cannot achieve acceptable alignment, stability, and congruency).

Preoperative Evaluation

The "site of pain" when specifically asked to locate site of pain, "one-finger test" [patient pointing out with a finger rather than putting his whole hand on the anterior part of knee ("knee grab")] are reliable examination findings. History of night pain/rest pain must be specifically asked for.

Standing anteroposterior (AP), lateral, Rosenberg, and skyline X-rays (to assess tibiofemoral alignment and the grade of OA in all three compartments) and stress X-rays (under direct supervision of the surgical team) are radiographic prerequisites **(Fig. 6)**.

Postoperative Protocol

Postoperative, Robert-Jones compression bandage is applied over sutured and dressed surgical wound; that is removed after 24–48 hours. Intravenous (IV) antibiotics (cephalosporin + aminoglycoside) are usually continued for 24 hours, thereafter oral antibiotics for 2–3 days. Postoperative AP and lateral X-rays of the knee (that include the maximal possible femoral and tibial length) are ordered to evaluate

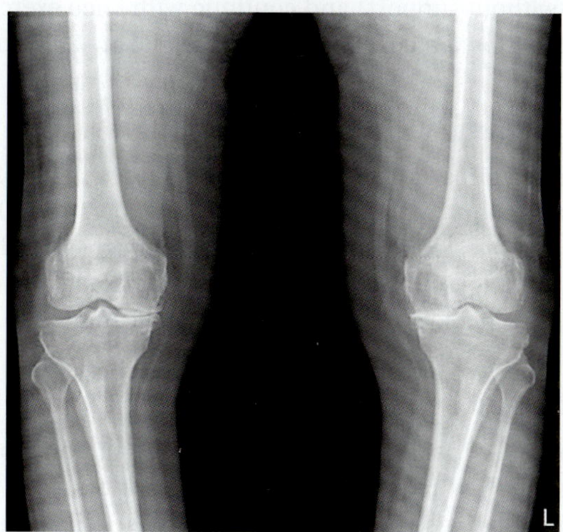

FIG. 6: X-ray depicting predominant medial compartmental osteoarthritis (OA) in both knees in a 79 years old male.

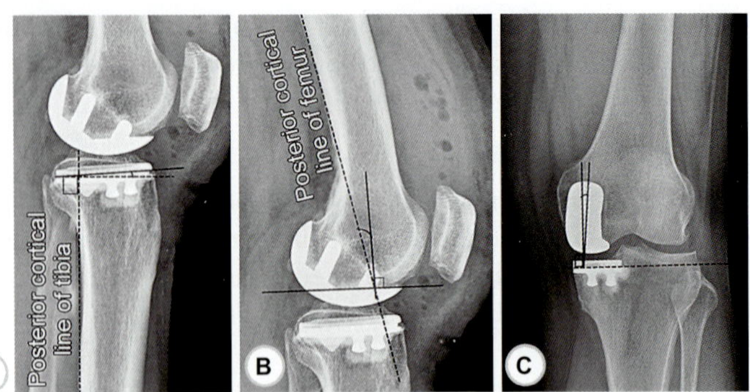

FIGS. 7A TO C: Radiographic evaluation of unicompartment knee arthroplasty (UKA). (A) Tibial component slope; (B) Femoral component sagittal alignment; and (C) Interprosthetic divergence.

alignment, component positioning and sizing, and to rule out patellar impingement, cement extrusion, or a fracture **(Fig. 7)**.

A multimodal approach of spinal anesthesia, atraumatic surgical technique, early mobilization, pneumatic devices (for compression), and low molecular weight heparin (LMWH) is used for deep vein thrombosis (DVT) prophylaxis. Mobilization is started with walker support on day 1, and by 2 weeks (staple removal), patients give up their supports and walk on their own, start stair climbing (initially with, later without support) and continue with knee exercises. Near complete functional recovery can be witnessed at ~2–3 months.

Complications

Early complications include inadequate pain relief (1–2%), DVT (1–5%), pulmonary embolism (<0.5%), infection (0.1–0.3%), pes anserinus bursitis, and femoral/tibial fractures; while loosening, subsidence, progression of arthritis in other compartments, poly wear and late infection, are known late complications.

Pros and Cons

Benefits of UKA include preservation of the quadriceps tendon, small incisions, less soft tissue dissection, less blood loss, and lower rate of complications (infection, pain, delayed rehabilitation, and reduced ROMs) and lesser hospital stay. Proprioception is better perceived, and patients have better subjective outcomes. Conversion to TKA is easier.

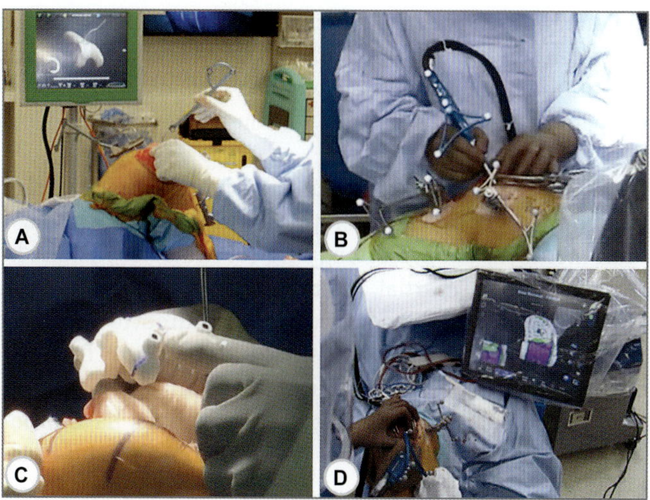

FIGS. 8A TO D: Newer tools in unicompartment knee arthroplasty (UKA) surgery that have made UKA more predictable. (A) Computer-navigated UKA; (B and D) Robotic-assisted UKA; (C) Patient-specific instrumentation (PSI).

Despite these advantages, potential pitfalls exist. These include improper exposure, soft tissue trauma (forceful retraction), improper implant positioning, and hence early failure. Concerns regarding survivability, patient selection, and ideal bearing design exist, though use of navigation/robotic assistance/patient-specific instrumentation has minimized the outliers **(Figs. 8A to D)**.

Conclusion

The superior functional outcomes and improved survivorship have led to the resurgence of UKA in the past decade. Contraindications are more well defined, limiting this surgery to either the "first arthroplasty" in younger patients or the "last arthroplasty" in very elderly carefully selected patients. With optimal surgical technique and use of technology, the survivability of UKA prostheses can be ensured.

PATELLOFEMORAL JOINT ARTHROPLASTY

Isolated patellofemoral osteoarthritis (PFOA) is the cause of anterior knee pain in approximately 10–24% of patients >40 years. Isolated PFOA is more commonly found in females, due to a higher incidence of patellofemoral dysplasia. Patients report pain behind the knee cap during squatting, lunging, bike riding, stair walking, hill climbing, sitting with the knee flexed for prolonged periods, and when rising from a seated position. In contrast, walking on level ground is rarely affected.

Initial treatment consists of activity modification, analgesics, weight reduction, physical therapy, bracing, patella taping, and injection therapy. Joint preserving surgical strategies include lateral release/lengthening, partial lateral facetectomy, chondroplasty, microfracture, mosaicplasty, autologous chondrocyte implantation, and anteromedial tibial tuberosity transfer with the goal of optimizing load-distribution and improving patellar alignment and tracking. Unfortunately, none of these procedures have produced reliable long-term results and are typically considered for patients aged <40 years. Patellofemoral joint arthroplasty (PFJA) is an option to address PFOA when the nonoperative or joint preserving management has failed, here intraoperative findings reveal the extensive patellofemoral degeneration **(Fig. 9)**.

Evolution of Implants

McKeever's initial design in 1955 used a Vitallium prosthesis to resurface the patella. Similar metal patellar arthroplasty designs were also developed by Insall and Worrell. In the late 1970s, the first generation of a complete PFJA using a polyethylene patellar resurfacing component and a metal trochlea was described. The poor results reported with these first-generation designs (Lubinus, Richards I, II, and III) led many surgeons to abandon this procedure.

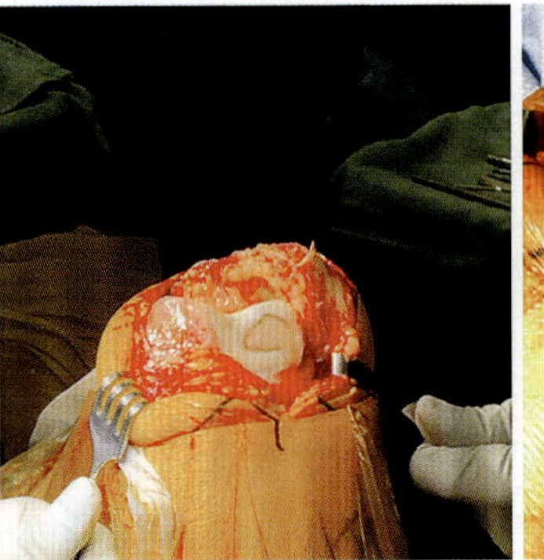
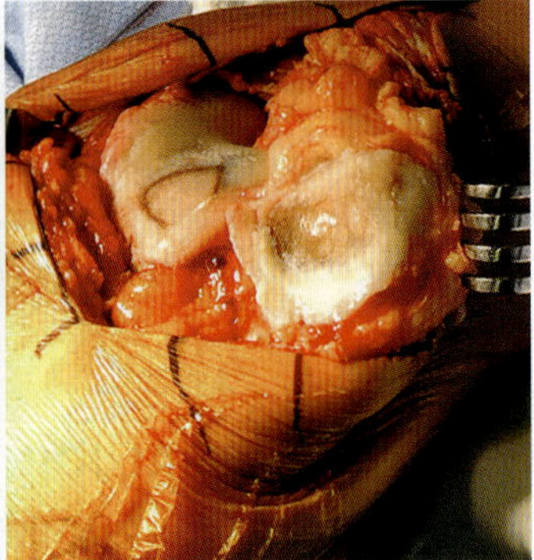

FIG. 9: Intraoperative picture showing extensive degeneration of patellofemoral joint.

Newer designs (onlay and inlay) have a wider trochlear component, longer proximal anterior flange, and more conforming radius of curvature, and use a central/offset dome shaped all poly patellar component, like the Avon (developed in 1996) **(Fig. 10)**.

Indications and Contraindications

Typical indications are patients with isolated symptomatic PFOA, with trochlear dysplasia, bone-on-bone (Iwano 4) PFOA, without significant malalignment and in the absence of risk factors for developing progressive tibiofemoral OA. PFJA can be considered in patients of 40–65 years old **(Fig. 11)**.

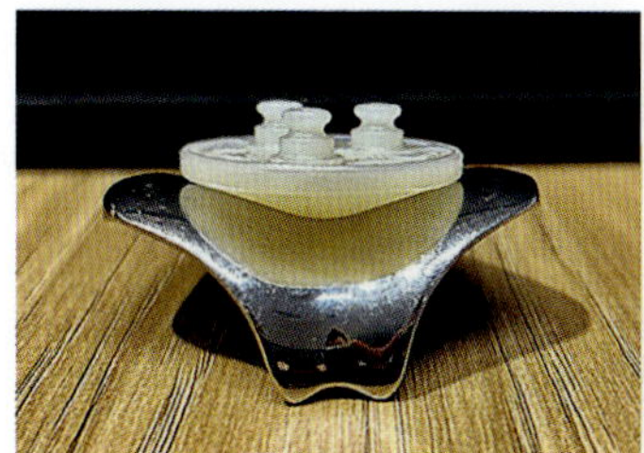
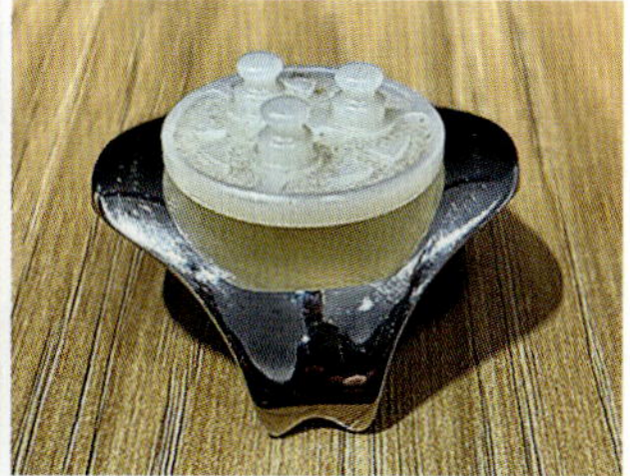

FIG. 10: Patellofemoral implant design: The Avon (Stryker) patellofemoral joint arthroplasty (PFJA) prosthesis.

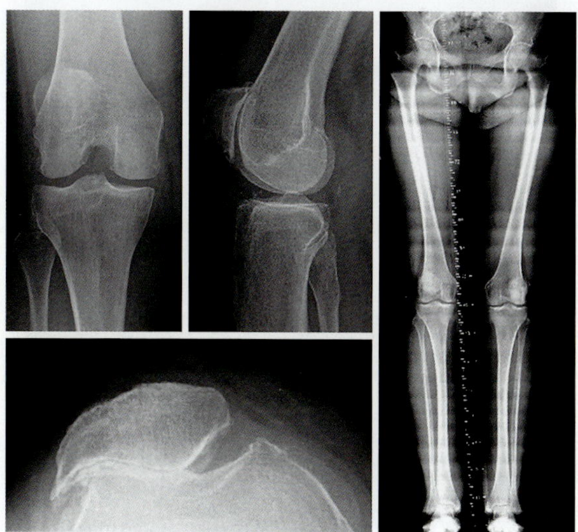

FIG. 11: Isolated symptomatic right isolated patellofemoral osteoarthritis (PFOA), trochlear dysplasia, and bone-on-bone (Iwano 4) osteoarthritis (OA).

Contraindications include tibiofemoral OA, systemic inflammatory disease, Iwano stages I/II, flexion contracture of >10° (associated with poorer outcomes), patella baja [Caton-Deschamps Index (CDI) <0.8]. Relative contraindications include a high knee flexion, distal femoral osteopenia, limb malalignment (>5° valgus and >3° varus).

Preoperative Evaluation

Clinical examination reveals patellofemoral crepitus, pain during active ROM, a positive Rabot sign, and quadriceps weakness. Varying degrees of lateral patella tilt and maltracking are usually found.

Pros and Cons

Common arguments in favor of PFJA are that it is a quicker procedure and recovery, bone sparing with more optimal postoperative knee kinematics **(Fig. 12)**.

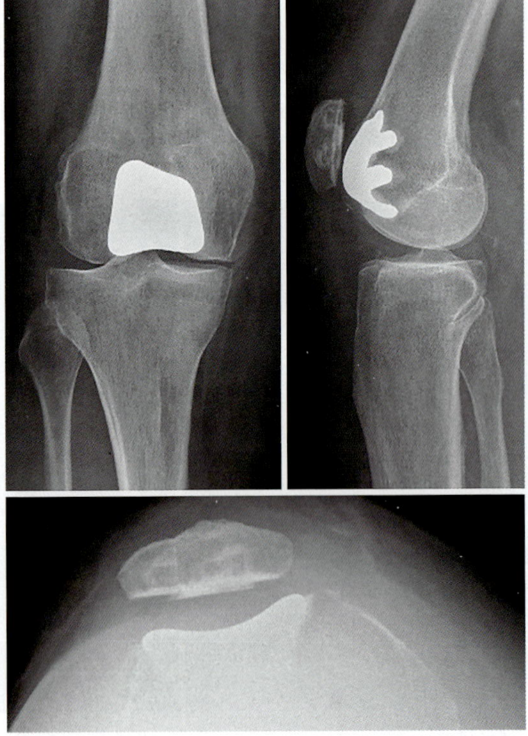

FIG. 12: Postoperative X-rays of right patellofemoral arthroplasty.

It is also technically easier to revise to a TKA (when needed). However, there are higher rate of revisions after PFJA (thus lower survival rates in national registries).

Conclusion

Patient selection remains crucial for the success of PFJA. Robotically assisted PFJA may allow for more precise implant positioning; however, research is required to determine if will translate into improved clinical outcomes.

BICOMPARTMENTAL KNEE ARTHROPLASTY

There is an increasing focus in providing patient specific procedures (with preservation of the cruciate ligaments) in knee arthroplasty so as to maintain normal knee kinematics. Bicompartmental knee arthroplasty (BCA), also known as combined partial knee arthroplasty (CPKA) has been gaining interest due to improved implant design with better clinical outcomes and survival rates.

Evolution of Implants

Initial BCAs utilized a linked monolithic prosthesis, associated with higher complication and revision rates (attributed to the difficulties with sizing and positioning of the femoral component, tibial subsidence, and tibial tray fracture) which ultimately led to the recall of the Journey Deuce prosthesis (Smith and Nephew Inc., Memphis, TN, US) by the USFDA in 2010. We now have 3D printed customized patient-specific instrumentation and implants, leading to improved results.

Primary Bicompartmental Knee Arthroplasty

Primary BCA may provide a potential alternative treatment option in those with bicompartmental disease (medial and lateral, medial and patellofemoral, lateral and patellofemoral arthritis). Medial tibiofemoral arthritis and PFJA arthritis is the most common combination and the most commonly performed BCA. Garner et al. recently developed a classification for combined partial knee arthroplasty (CPKA) [bi-unicondylar arthroplasty (Bi-UKA), medial bicompartmental arthroplasty (BCA-M), lateral bicompartmental arthroplasty (BCA-L)] **(Fig. 13)**.

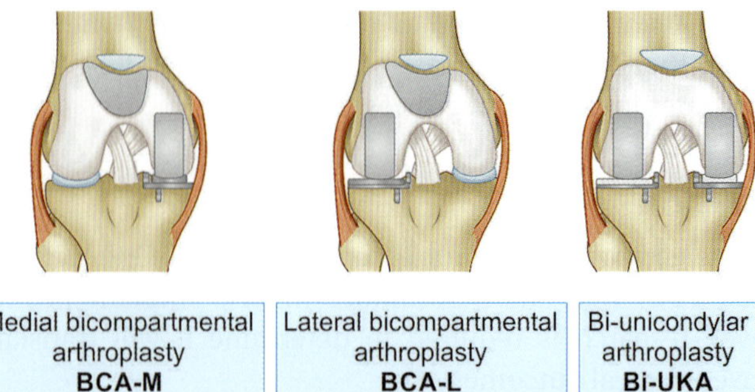

FIG. 13: Classification of combined partial knee arthroplasty.

Pros and Cons

Advantages include preservation of bone and cruciate ligaments and improvements in anterior-posterior stability and extensor efficiency. Concerns (more so in UKA to BCA conversions) include knee balancing, subsidence, loosening, and disease progression. It must be realized that not all patients are suitable for conversion of UKA to BCA (raised BMI, multiple medical comorbidities). Rates of re-revision in UKA to BCA vary with some papers reporting rates of 17% compared to 7% in UKA to TKA.

Conclusion

There may be a role for BCA as an alternative treatment option for bicompartmental OA in a certain subset of younger patients with a desire to a faster recovery, preservation of normal knee kinematics, who want to postpone a TKA. However, *the procedure is technically demanding, and the surgeon should be a high-volume practitioner, proficient in performing UKA and PFJA.*

Patient specific instrumentation (PSI) and robotic-assisted surgery may have a greater part to play in addressing some of the difficulties encountered with the positioning, sizing, and alignment of the BCA implants.

BICRUCIATE RETAINING TOTAL KNEE ARTHROPLASTY

Despite technical advancement and a 20-year survival rate exceeding 90%, approximately 20% of patients nowadays remain unsatisfied after surgery. It is believed that this dissatisfaction may be overcome by improving the abnormal kinematics and proprioceptive instability reported after sacrificing the ACL in current TKA designs [whether posterior-stabilized (PS) or posterior cruciate-retaining (CR)].

Bicruciate retaining (BCR) TKA was developed to mimic knee biomechanics, through ACL preservation.

Evolution of Implants

The first example of cruciate-sparing prosthesis was developed by Gunston in 1960, the "Polycentric Knee", an implant was composed by two semicircular cemented femoral sliding tracks with two distinct cemented fixed tibial components. Subsequently, the Mayo clinic team created the "Geometric" knee prosthesis composed of two femoral components linked with a crossbar (to retain both cruciates) and a unique poly with an anterior tibial island bridge.

Modern advances in technology have resulted in the introduction of two models of BCR-TKA [Vanguard XP Total Knee System (Zimmer Biomet, Warsaw, IN, United States) and Journey II XR (Smith and Nephew plc, Watford, United Kingdom)] **(Fig. 14)**.

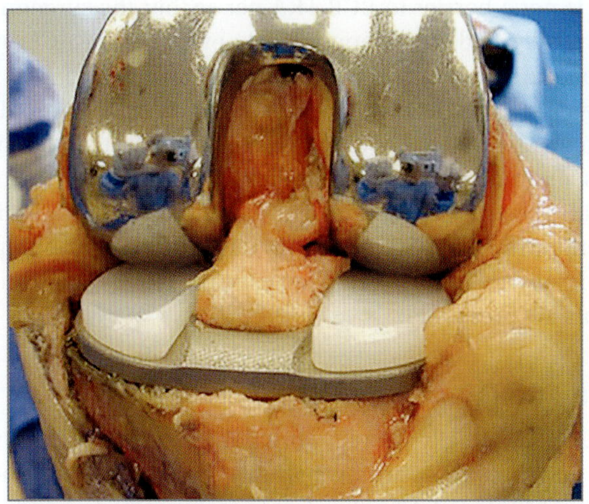

FIG. 14: A BCR-TKA prosthesis (Journey-II XR), showing preservation of intercondylar notch and both cruciates.

(BCR: bicruciate retaining; TKA: total knee arthroplasty)

Table 1: Indications and relative contraindications summary for BCR-TKA.

Indications	*Relative contraindication*
High-demand patients	Low-demand patients
End-stage bi- or tricompartmental knee OA	Severe coronal malalignment (>15°)
Coronal malalignment <15°	Inflammatory arthritis
ACL integrity	ACL mucoid degeneration/absence
Clinical assessment (Lachman, anterior drawer test, and pivot shift test)	Relevant preoperative reduction of ROM (>10°)
Intraoperative assessment	
Minimal ROM reduction (<5/10°)	

(ACL: anterior cruciate ligament; BCR: bicruciate retaining; OA: osteoarthritis; ROM: range of motion; TKA: total knee arthroplasty)

Indications and Contraindications

There is a significant overlap between recent UKA and BCR-TKA indications **(Table 1)**.

Age is not a barrier to BCR-TKA per se, but the surgeon should preoperatively and/or intraoperatively evaluate the ACL integrity, the coronal alignment, and ROM limitations.

Severe (>15°) coronal malalignment is a contraindication. Inadequate research exists to understand the effect of inflammatory arthritis and mucoid degeneration on ACL integrity to permit BCR-TKA. It also seems appropriate to initially limit BCR-TKA indications to patients with minimal reduction (<10°) in ROM as preoperative motion issues are more likely to persist after TKA if both the cruciate ligaments are preserved.

Pros and Cons

The BCR-TKA ideally would combine the expected advantage of UKA in terms of restoring natural knee kinematics and long-term survival rates of TKA. Surgery is technically demanding, with failures occurring mostly due to poly wear, aseptic loosening of the components, and infection.

Conclusion

The renewed interest in BCR-TKA is mainly rooted on component design improvement and biomechanical and kinematical studies, that corroborate the possible significant advantage that retention of cruciate ligaments can offer rather than high-quality long-term clinical trials.

Chapter 26

Technology Today

Technology today encompasses the use of computer-assisted surgery (CAS), robotic-assisted surgery (RAS), and patient-specific instruments and implants (PSI) using three-dimensional (3D) printing technology. Some of these trends [like computer-assisted/navigated total knee arthroplasty (TKA)] have been modified/upgraded to include other technology (use of robotics and 3D printed implants with PSI) and are slowly gaining traction as the standard of care.

COMPUTER-ASSISTED SURGERY—TOTAL KNEE ARTHROPLASTY

In TKA, component alignment influences knee function and implant longevity. Conventional jig-based TKA utilizes preoperative X-rays, intraoperative anatomical landmarks, and manually positioned alignment jigs to guide bone resections and implant positioning. This is associated with the risk of poor reproducibility, possible soft tissue iatrogenic injuries, and limited intraoperative data on gap measurements or ligamentous tensioning, leading to alignment and balancing errors. CAS permits measurement of all the steps of the TKA procedure with a high degree (error <1 mm, $<1°$) of accuracy.

The key features of CAS TKA are 3D reconstruction (bone morphing for comprehensive anatomical information with/without preoperative diagnostic imaging), true implant integration (adaptation of software and instruments to specific implants), pre- and intraoperative 3D planning to optimize implant position, alignment (before any cuts are made), advanced kinematic analysis (inbuilt software demonstrating real-time knee kinematics), intraoperative verification and updation of bone resections, and finally providing an automatic therapy report (for scientific data collection and documentation).

Evolution

The first computer-navigated TKA was reportedly performed in 1997, the early system consisting of a computer, optical localizer, and arrays mounted with light emitting diodes (LEDs) which could be attached to bones and surgical instruments to aid in the desired placement of cutting blocks. This technology has undergone extensive validation and upgrades over the years.

The essential components of a computer navigation system are the computer system, trackers/arrays, and the localizer/camera **(Figs. 1A to C)**.

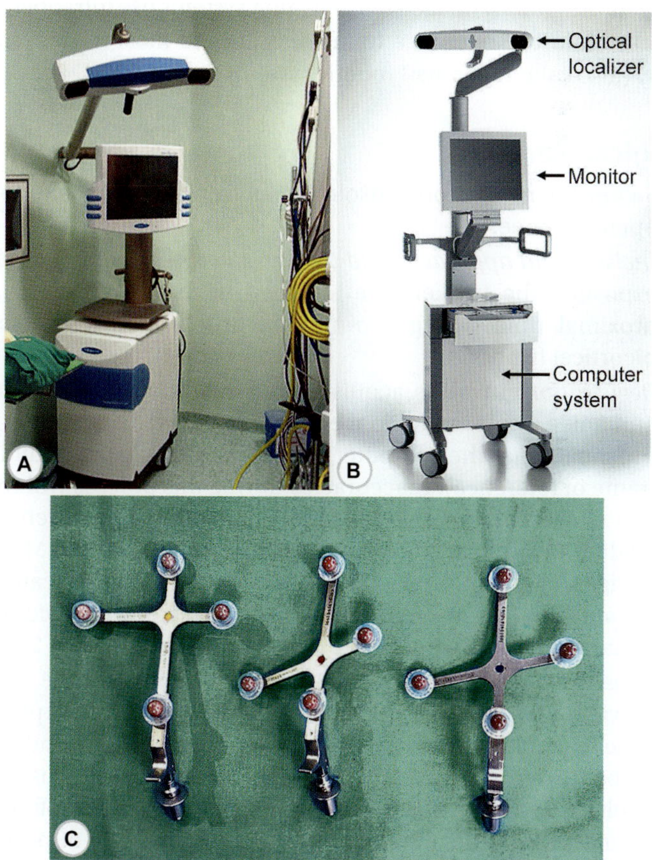

FIGS. 1A TO C: (A) Contemporary computer-assisted surgery (CAS) system; (B) Its main parts highlighted; (C) Passive arrays with reflective "optical" spheres.

During surgery, trackers are attached to the bones, surgical instruments, or a probe. They can be "passive" in the form of reflective spheres, or "active" with LEDs. The localizer (or camera) receives reflected (passive tracker) or active (active tracker) signals from the trackers to determine their spatial orientation. The most used localizers are *optical* localizers (requiring "line of sight"). *Electromagnetic* systems do not need "line of sight" (they have a receiver that can detect signals from the trackers).

Types of Computer-assisted Surgery

The CAS/navigation systems can be large-console navigation systems (image-based or imageless) or accelerometer-based handheld navigation systems. Imageless navigation systems use intraoperative data to build the reference frame and are the most used systems today (also called "passive" robotic systems).

Surgical Workflow

- *Setup:* The navigation console is usually placed opposite to the operated knee.
- *Incision and approach (and tracker placement)*: After standard exposure, the trackers are attached to the distal femur and proximal tibia (using two-pin unicortical or a single-screw bicortical fixation).
- *Registration:* Involves acquisition of centers of the hip, knee, and ankle joints, and surface mapping of the distal femur and proximal tibia (the computer system uses this data to build the frame of reference). Inaccuracies during this process will result in incorrect data being displayed by the system, eventually leading to surgical errors ("garbage in, garbage out"). Modern navigation systems have built-in redundancies which can alert the surgeon if there is a significantly large error while acquiring certain landmarks during the registration process **(Fig. 2)**.
- *Bone morphing:* Once the registration is completed, the system provides information about limb alignment and joint morphology which the surgeon can use to determine the orientation and depth of bone resections, titrate soft-tissue releases, and customize implant position to obtain desired alignment and soft tissue balance. One can control the orientation and depth of proximal tibial and distal femoral resections, adjust femoral size, and set femoral (and even tibial) rotation, permitting 3D customization of implant position based on surgeon's preference **(Figs. 3A and B)**.

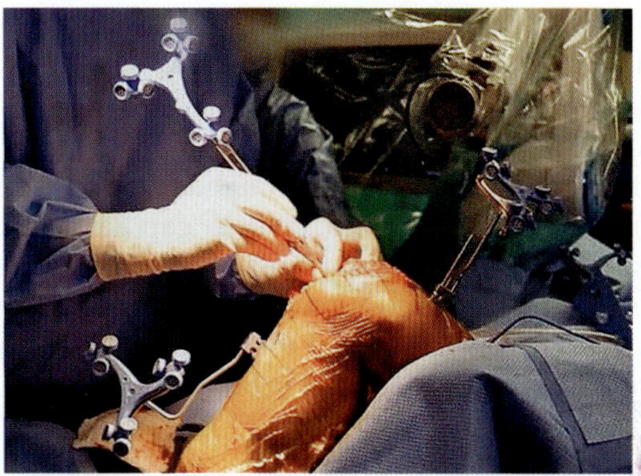

FIG. 2: Intraoperative picture showing placement of arrays and registration process.

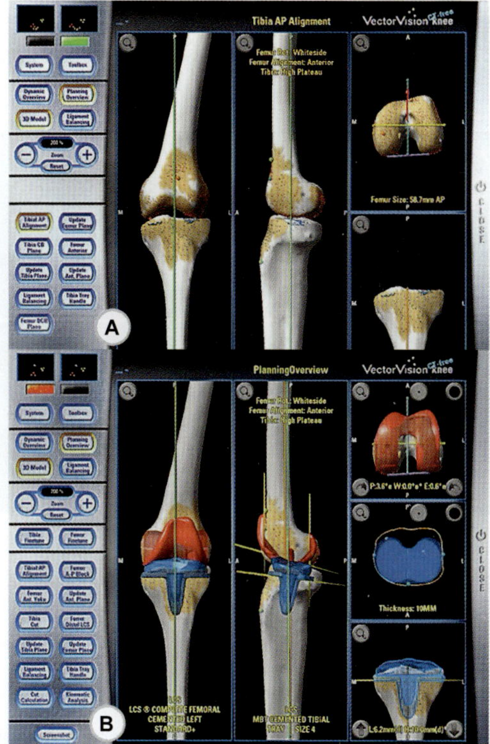

FIGS. 3A AND B: Computer screen image during surgery: (A) Rendering 3D model; and (B) Providing information about size and positioning of femoral and tibial components.

- *Bone resections:* The surgeon carries out the bone resections according to the pre- and intraoperative plan.
- *Verification:* One can then verify the cuts (and recut, if required). Most contemporary systems also provide data about joint kinematics and balance throughout knee range of motion (ROM) before and after bone cuts. If "gap balancing" protocol is chosen, medial and lateral knee joint gaps in extension and 90° flexion are displayed (which the surgeon can use to plan soft tissue releases and adjust the femoral implant position to achieve desired alignment and balance) **(Figs. 4A to E)**.

Handheld Navigation

Handheld navigation works with a system of sensors which are attached to cutting guides or bones to aid in the placement of cutting blocks in a desired position. They were launched with the aim of overcoming some of the drawbacks of large-console systems, e.g., KneeAlign 2 (KA2) (OrthAlign, Inc.; Aliso Viejo, CA) **(Fig. 5)**.

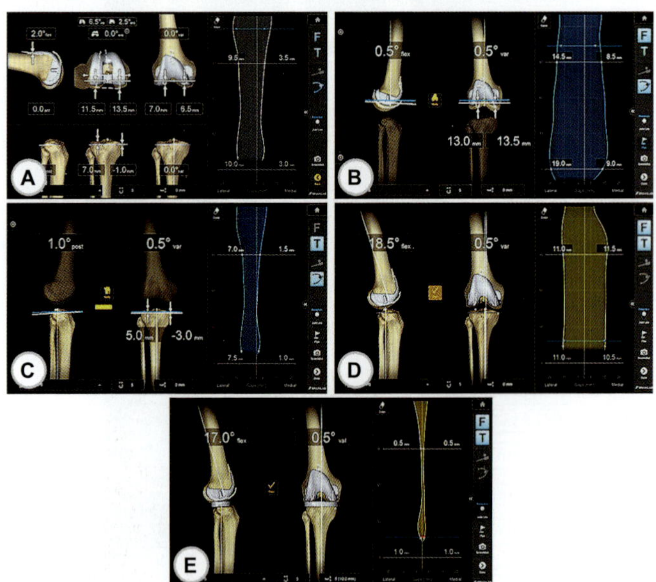

FIGS. 4A TO E: Navigational workflow. (A) Planning bony resection and expected gaps; (B) Distal femoral resection and expected extension gap; (C) Tibial resection and expected flexion and extension gaps; (D) Gap assessment with the trial components; and (E) Secondary gap assessment with tibial poly insert.

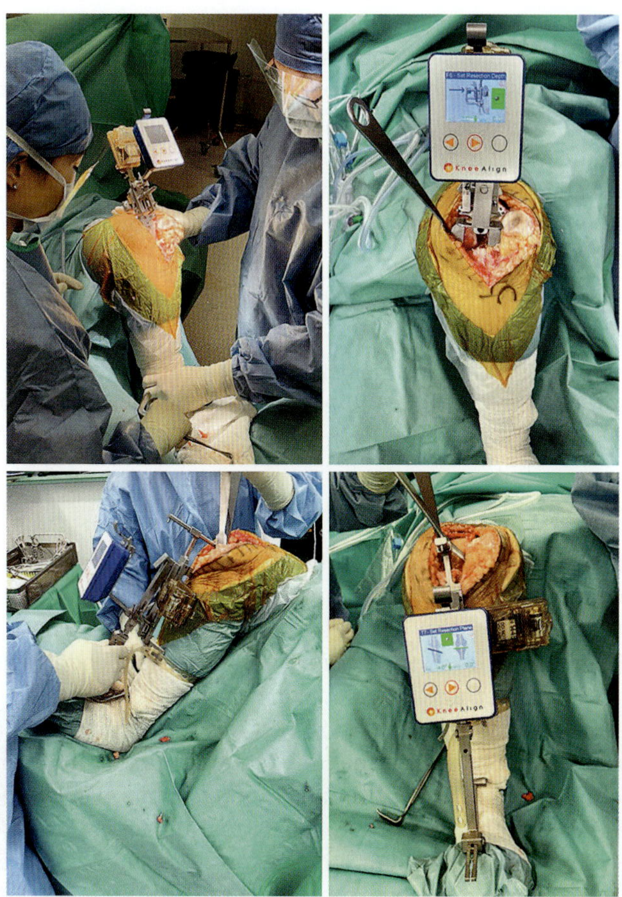

FIG. 5: Intraoperative photos using handheld navigation for proximal tibial and distal femoral cuts.

Handheld CAS systems have the advantages of having no initial setup cost, no "line of sight" problems associated with optical tracking, no pin sites (pinless), and reduced surgical time. However, these systems do not provide information about soft-tissue tension and cannot aid in setting component rotations. Also, as the components are of single use, there is a per patient cost involved.

Pros and Cons

Certain situations where the utility of navigation cannot be overemphasized are in patients with extra-articular deformities of the femur or tibia, retained hardware in the distal femur, and knees with ipsilateral long stem total hip arthroplasty (THAs). Cost (both for initial setup and recurring), pin track issues (infection, fractures) and learning curve-related complications are issues, and persist with the advancement to robotic-assisted TKA. Navigated TKA improves implant alignment, however, saw blade thickness, deflection, and cutting guide motion may lead to final bone cuts differing from planned resections.

Conclusion

The superiority of computer navigation over conventional TKA in improving *accuracy* is well-established. The next step involves improving *precision* of the cuts (robotic-assisted TKA closes this gap).

ROBOTIC-ASSISTED SURGERY

Actual/real-time saw blade errors (thickness, deflection, and cutting guide motion) may lead to suboptimal component alignment. This error is reduced dramatically by the concurrent use of a robotic bone cutting tool that provides *precision* (uses real-time feedback to the user of the planned and executed bone cuts).

Robotic-assisted surgery (RAS) TKA also uses computer software to convert anatomical information [X-rays, computed tomography (CT) scans, or anatomic landmarks] into a virtual patient-specific 3D reconstruction of the knee. This virtual model is then used to plan optimal bone resection, implant positioning, bone coverage, and limb alignment based on the patient's unique anatomy, and the robotic bone cutting tool executes this plan to precision.

Evolution

The first surgical robots were used in prostate cancer surgery (1985) and neurosurgery (1988) to guide biopsies. In 2002, the da Vinci Robot System® (Intuitive Surgical, Sunnyvale, CA, USA) initiated a new concept of robotic surgery, transforming both medical practice and learning. The first available orthopedic robotic system in TKA was the Robodoc® (THINK Surgical Inc., Fremont, California, USA), introduced in 1992.

Robots in Total Knee Arthroplasty

Depending on the orthopedic surgeon's external control, the robots are classified as passive, fully active, or semi-active systems. Further, robotic systems can be image-based (X-rays/CT) or imageless (only rely on intraoperative points) for registration; and are closed (only one implant system can be used with the robot), or open (where any/different implant system can be used with the said robot) systems.

- *Passive:* Passive systems work under the continuous and direct control of the surgeon. The robotic systems delineate patient anatomical data and provide objective real-time feedback on guide placement for optimal bone resection and implant placement. However, the robot does not actively control or restrain the surgeon in performing any aspect of the procedure. Navigated or CAS TKA are passive robotic systems.
- *Fully active:* The surgeon performs the surgical approach, places retractors to protect the soft tissues, and secures the limb to a fixed device, and finally, the robotic device executes the planned bone resections autonomously. However, the surgeon can check and deactivate it in case of emergency [ROBODOC (THINK Surgical Inc., Fremont, California, USA) and ROSA (Zimmer–Biomet, Warsaw, IN, USA) (active, closed platform, X-ray image-based)]. The ROSA Knee System® is different, because this robotic system converts two-dimensional knee X-rays into a 3D patient-specific bone model. A virtual plan on implant positioning and ligament balancing is created, robotically positioned cutting block jigs then guide the surgeon to manually perform the bone cuts through the cutting blocks **(Figs. 6A to C)**.
- *Semi-active:* The robotic arm has visual, tactile, and audio feedback that help the surgeon to control the force and direction of saw blade/burr action within haptic boundaries (confines of the femoral and tibial bone resection windows). The patient's limb is usually secured within a mobile leg holder boot, rapid or jerky movements deactivate the robotic device and limit iatrogenic bone and soft tissue injury. These include the Mako (Stryker Ltd, Kalamazoo, MI, USA) (semi-active, closed platform, and CT image-based) **(Figs. 7A and B)** and CORI (Smith & Nephew, Andover, Texas, USA) (semi-active, open platform, and imageless) **(Figs. 8A to C)** among others.

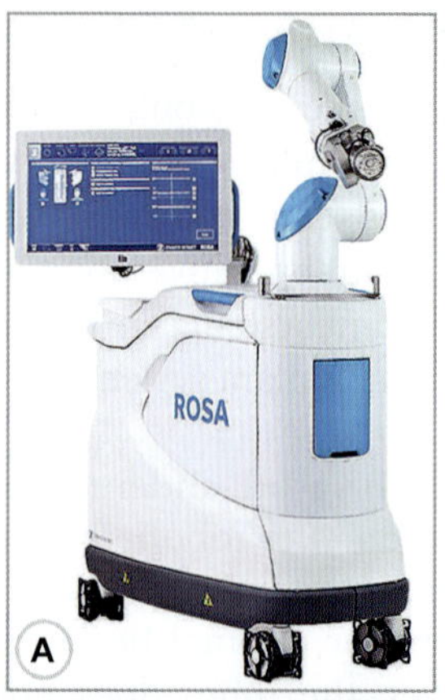

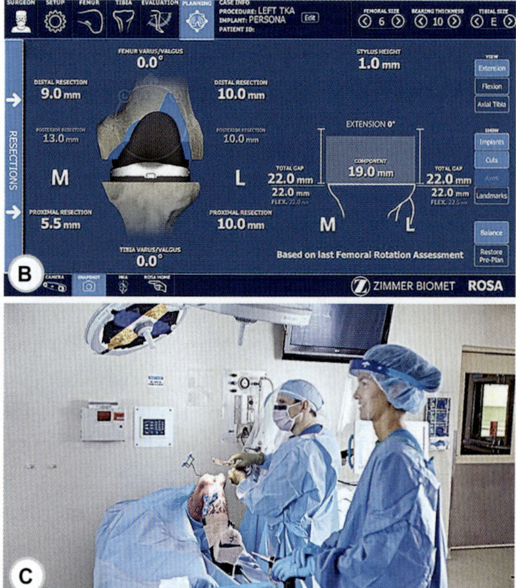

FIGS. 6A TO C: (A) ROSA system for TKA; (B) Software for preoperative and intraopeartive planning based on implant positioning and soft tissue tensioning; and (C) ROSA arm attaching cutting block for femoral cut.

(TKA: total knee arthroplasty)

Surgical Workflow

Five distinct stages include the following:

1. *Preoperative radiography:* Plain X-rays/CT scans of the knee are used to create a virtual 3D reconstruction of the patient's native knee anatomy.

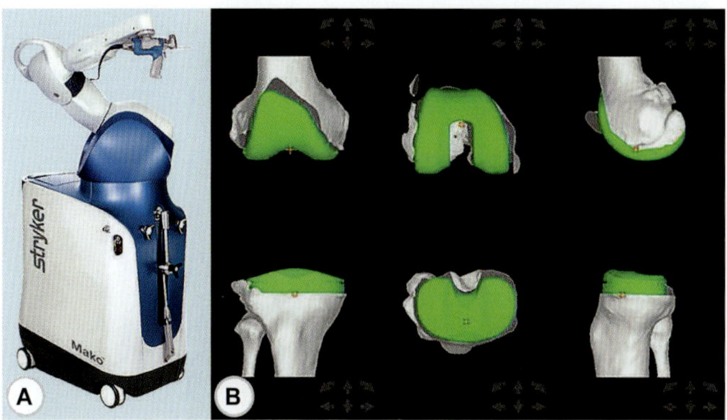

FIGS. 7A AND B: (A) Mako robot for TKA; and (B) Mako's computer software for preoperative templating.

(TKA: total knee arthroplasty)

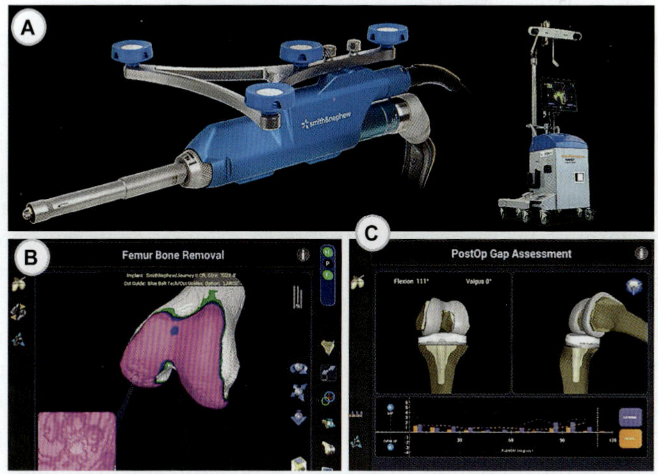

FIGS. 8A TO C: (A) CORI/Navio robot and its computer software for TKA; (B) Burring window for femoral component preparation; and (C) Intraoperative gap assessment with trial implants.

(TKA: total knee arthroplasty)

2. *Planning:* The surgeon (and robotic engineer) uses this virtual model to plan optimal implant positioning, alignment, and sizing. Computer software calculate femoral and tibial bone resection windows for accomplishing this surgical plan with a high level of precision.

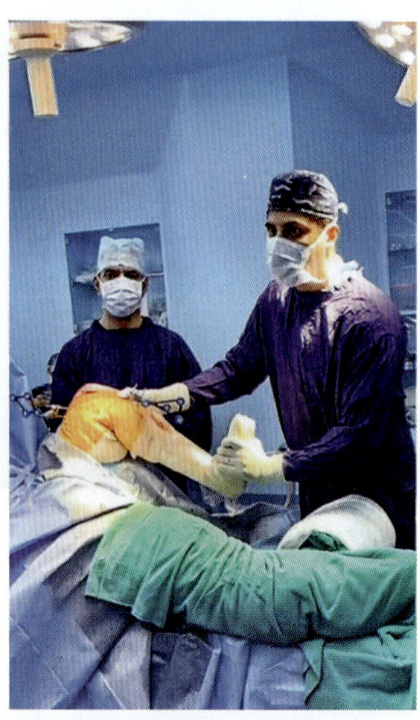

FIG. 9: Intraoperative image showing assessment of balance in range of motion (ROM).

3. *Intraoperative steps:* Tibial and femoral array positioning, intraoperative bone registration, and verification of bony landmarks are done. In imageless systems, registration is performed by mapping the patient's osseous anatomy onto a generic virtual model of the knee, with implant position and bone resection plans performed intraoperative in real-time **(Fig. 9)**.

   In CT-based robotic knee systems, a patient-specific knee model is created preoperative, and osseous anatomy is mapped intraoperative to reconfirm the bone geometry. The system can be set for a "measured resection" or "gap balancing" technique, offering the possibility to modify the position and eventually the size of the component on the 3D virtual model. A virtual balancing is then performed. When all knee positions are registered, a gap balancing graph will show the joint stability for each captured flexion position **(Fig. 9)**.

   Once the joint is virtually balanced, the robotic arm is correctly positioned, and the next stage begins.
4. *Robot-assisted bone resections:* The surgeon uses the robotic device to perform the bone resections within the preplanned boundaries of the femoral and tibial bone windows **(Fig. 10)**.

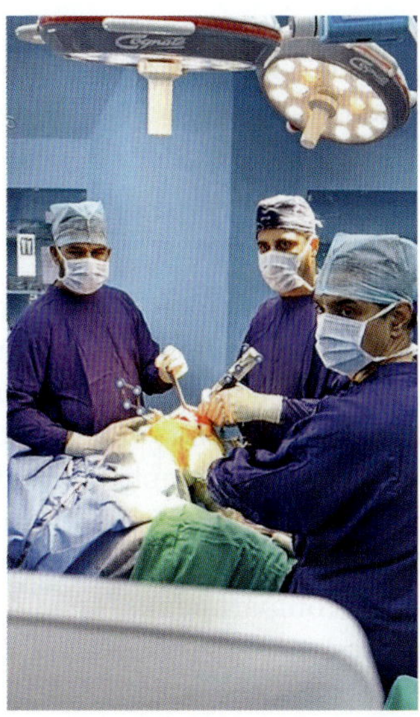

FIG. 10: Intraoperative image showing use of robotic burr for femoral preparation.

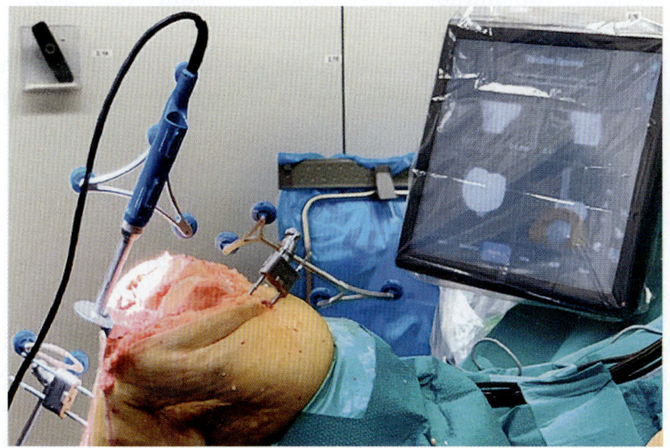

FIG. 11: Intraoperative image showing computer screen and bone cut verification.

5. *Assessment and check:* Optical motion capture technology is used to reassess intraoperative flexion and extension gaps, joint stability, range of movement, and limb alignment **(Fig. 11)**. The surgeon can then perform live on-table modifications to bone

resection, implant positioning, and fine-tune soft tissue releases to achieve the desired bone coverage, component positioning, knee kinematics, and limb alignment. All these can be rechecked after implantation, and the obtained data recorded.

Pros and Cons

Robotic-assisted TKA provides improved accuracy *and precision* of bone cuts and implant positioning. Limitations include the initial economic investment, additional radiation exposure for the patients (in image-based platforms), increased operative times, and increased risk of short-term complications during the learning curve (i.e., superficial infection, iatrogenic fractures, and common peroneal injury). Different application systems need to be purchased for THA, TKA, and unicompartmental knee arthroplasty (UKA), leading to more expenses.

Conclusion

The surgeon uses an intraoperative robotic device to execute the preoperative (or intraoperative) planned bone resections and implant position, and an intraoperative robotic device executes this plan with a high level of precision, but whether this translates into improved patient-reported outcomes and long-term survivorship is still a matter of debate.

PERSONALIZED TOTAL KNEE ARTHROPLASTY (USING PATIENT-SPECIFIC IMPLANTS/ INSTRUMENTS AND 3D PRINTING)

Anatomical studies have shown considerable gender and ethnicity related variations of knee anatomy, which causes a substantial incidence of femoral component overhang and alignment issues when using over the shelf noncustomized prosthesis. Advancements in research and technology over the past decades have accelerated the transition from standardized or "mean value" medicine toward personalized or "precision" medicine, where medical decisions, treatments, and products are tailored to each patient depending on their predicted response and risk factors.

Personalized TKA involves the adaptation of specific parameters or features, to match the prearthritic anatomy and/or restore native kinematics. The personalized parameters (viz., coronal, sagittal, or rotational alignment, joint line obliquity, flexion/extension gaps, and condylar curvature) are used concurrently with the personalizing tools (3D imaging, preoperative planning software, PSI, navigation, and/or robotics).

Evolution

Smith–Peterson took molds of the femoral condyles to produce personalized "resurfacing" implants in the 1940s. In the 1970s, Freeman and Insall introduced "mechanical" implants requiring planar bone resections. The popularization of personalized TKA is propelled by three main drivers, the fall of the dogma of mechanical alignment, a greater appreciation of the variability of knee phenotypes, and evolution of diagnostic, planning, and assistive technologies.

Availability of custom instruments and jigs (3D printed HMWPE) **(Fig. 12)** designed to fit onto individual bony anatomy, and custom implants (3D printed metal implants that match the contour and size of the patient's native bony anatomy) has led to the emergence of personalized TKA surgery.

Functional Alignment

Various authors recently proposed functional alignment (FA) as a technique that aims to reconstruct the 3D constitutional

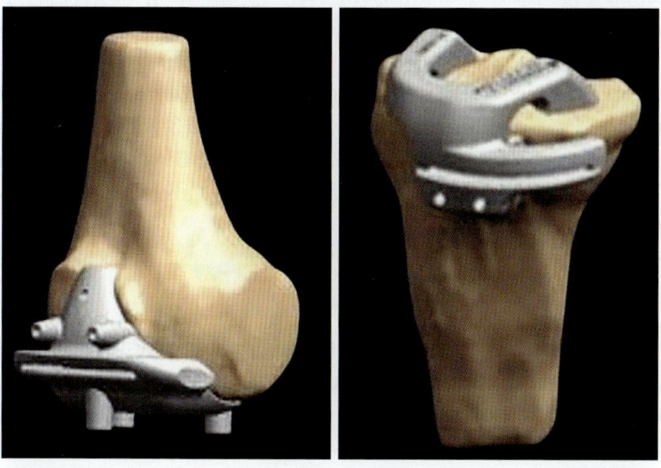

FIG. 12: 3D printed patient-specific jigs for distal femoral and proximal tibial cuts.

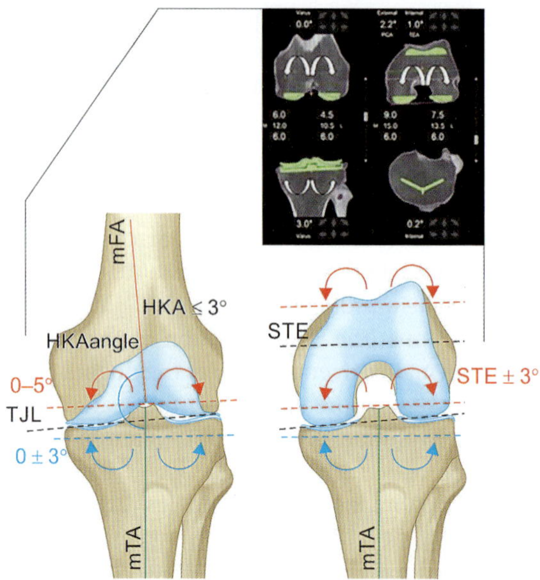

FIG. 13: Functional alignment, confirmed with robotic assistance.

alignment of the knee, whilst maintaining the adapted soft tissue envelope. This they found was possible with the aid of a robotic system. FA differs from other kinematic alignment (KA) alignment techniques (kinematic, restricted kinematic, inverse kinematic, adjusted mechanical alignment, etc.) by defining targets for joint height, obliquity, and balanced gaps throughout the ROM along with objective soft tissue laxity endpoints. Safe boundaries [*hip-knee-ankle (HKA) axis:* 6° varus to 3° valgus; *femoral component:* 6° valgus to 3° varus; *tibial component:* 6° varus to 3° valgus; combined component flexion<10°, and *femoral rotation:* 6° valgus to 6° varus] are defined, within which modifications are allowed to achieve a balanced knee **(Fig. 13)**.

3D Printing

3D printing is the process of utilizing materials such as plastic, ceramic, or metals, to manufacture objects using 3D model data. 3D models have the potential to act as visual and tactile aids, allowing surgeons to study complex cases, plan preoperative (including implant sizing, quantity and type of graft needed, and bone cuts)

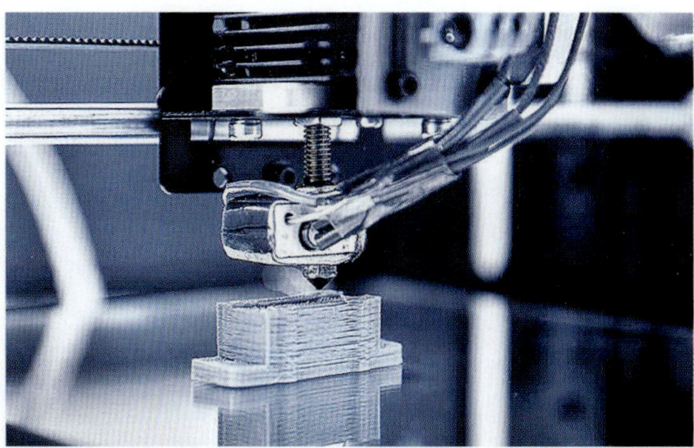

FIG. 14: 3D printer using additive manufacturing to print metallic shape.

and rehearse the procedure (to minimize intraoperative surprises and risks).

The 3D printing process produces objects using either layer-by-layer printing (using CAD software), or by additive manufacturing (AM) technology (material extrusion method). AM allows the fabrication of customized patient-specific implants based on their size, shape, and mechanical qualities. Materials used include ABS plastic, polylactic acid (PLA) (nylon), glass-filled polyamide, epoxy resins (epoxy resins), silver, titanium, steel, wax, photopolymers, poly carbonate (PC), cells, and hydrogels **(Fig. 14)**.

The femoral component made of Co-Cr is 3D printed using selective laser melting. Titanium-aluminum-vanadium alloy (Ti-6Al-4V) and conventional polyethylene are used to make the tibia and tibial implants, respectively **(Figs. 15A to F)**.

Pros and Cons

Personalized implants offer three distinct advantages: Optimization of bone-implant fit, decoupling of the patellofemoral from the tibiofemoral compartment, and restoration of native condylar curvature. Lower transfusion rates, lower adverse event rates, superior mechanical axis reproduction, and more consistent coronal alignment of the femoral component have been shown by some authors. It is unfortunately still unclear if we should restore all native anatomy and ligament laxity in TKA. The utility of patient-specific implants also remains unsubstantiated by the available literature.

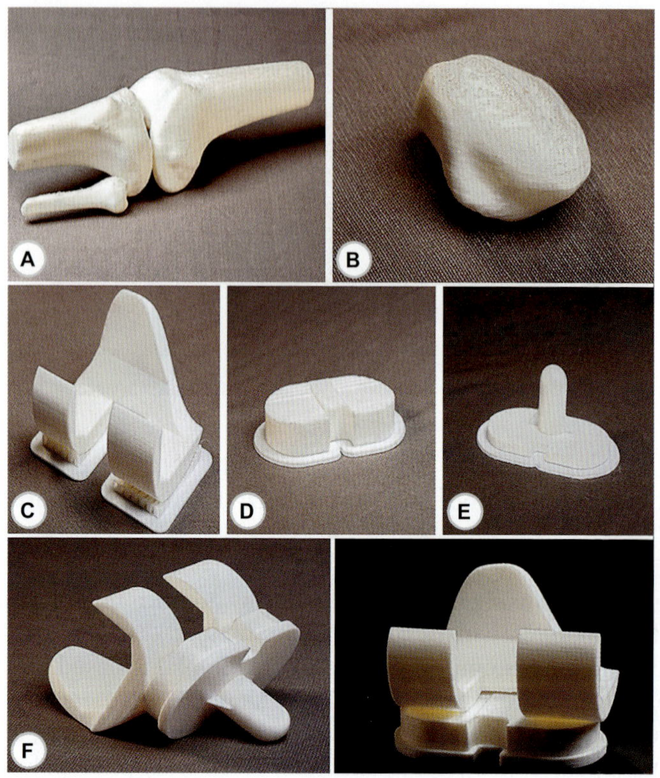

FIGS. 15A TO F: 3D printed prototypes. (A) Bones of the knee joint; (B) Patella; (C) Femoral implant; (D) Tibial insert liner; (E) Tibial tray; and (F) Knee implant assembly.

Conclusion

Custom/personalized implants might be a promising complement to a holistic solution for the problem of dissatisfaction following TKA. Using multiple alignment strategies (FA) and technology (3D printed implants, robot assistance), there is a strong possibility of improved outcomes.

Index

Page numbers followed by *f* refer to figure and *t* refer to table.

A

Accelerated physiotherapy protocol 110
Ahlback osteoarthritis stages 141*f*
Air filters 135
Alignment
  functional 167
  normal
    coronal 11
    rotational 13
    sagittal 12
  stability, and mobility check 58
  types of 11, 13
Allegretto unicompartment knee system 141*f*
Aminoglycoside 143
Anesthesia risk 35
Antibiotic-loaded cement 137
Anticoagulant
  antiplatelet aggregatory drugs 36
  chemoprophylaxis 121
  direct oral 114
  prophylaxis 119
Antiplatelet medication 132
Arrays, placement of 157*f*
Arthritic knee in
  flexion 85
  recurvatum 97
Arthritis
  altered anatomy in 10
  severity of 3
Arthrodesed knee 100
Arthrofibrosis 125
Arthroscopic joint debridement 138
Articular surface incongruity 27
Aseptic loosening 125
Attune tibial insert 17
Autologous chondrocyte implantation 138
Automatic therapy report 154

B

Bearing type 130
Betascrub 37
Biceps femoris 6
Bicompartmental knee arthroplasty 149
  evolution of implants 149
  primary 149
Biomechanics 74
Bleeding
  high risk of 121
  tendencies 132
Blood pressure 105
Body exhaust systems 136*f*
  use of 136
Bone cement
  defect managed with 92*f*
  tibial implant and tibial surface with 68*f*
Bone cuts 75, 80, 86, 97, 101, 127
  verification 165*f*
Bone defects 90*f*
  X-rays of 91*f*
Bone deficiencies 90
Bone grafting 94*f*
  defect managed with morselized impaction 93*f*
  multiple techniques for 91
Bone morphing 156
Bone preservation and revision 130
Bone resections 158
Bone-on-bone osteoarthritis 147*f*
Bony cortical rim 90

C

Caton-deschamps index 148
Cavitary defects 90
Cement 65, 130, 130*t*
  sets 69
  vacuum mixers 133
Cephalosporin 143
Ceramics 4
Chamfer cuts 58*f*
Charcot's joints 29, 30*f*
Compartmental knee arthroplasty 138
Component implantation 64
Compression stockings 109
Computer navigation system, essential components of 155
Computer-assisted surgery system 154, 155*f*
Computer-assisted surgery, types of 156
Condylar knee prosthesis, constrained 3*f*
Cortical bone, intact rim of 90
Custom instruments and jigs 167

D

da Vinci Robot System® 160
Deep dissection, standard approach 20*f*
Deep incision and approach 49
Deep medial collateral ligament 19
Deep vein thrombosis 35, 114, 121, 144
  chemoprophylaxis 115*f*
  incidence based on risk factor scores 116, 116*t*
  incidence of 131
  mechanical 107
  prevention of 114*f*
  prophylaxis 115*f*
    stockings for 107*f*
Deformity 43, 48
Detensioning stitch, modified 125*f*
Diabetes mellitus 137
Diathermy
  apparatus 32*f*
  machines 31
Distal femoral 138
  bone cut 51
  cut 53, 53*f*, 81*f*
    3D printed specific jigs for 167*f*
  cutting block 53*f*
Distal femur
  cutting block set 53*f*
  notch cutting jig on 57*f*
Dressing 71
Duocondylar knee 1

E

Electromagnetic systems 156
Electronic tourniquet 32*f*
Epicondyle slide osteotomy, medial 26
Epoxy resins 169
Erythrocyte sedimentation rate 125
Extensor hallucis longus 84
Extramedullary jig 51
Extramedullary tibial alignment jig, placement of 51*f*

F

Femoral and tibial bone resection 163
Femoral and tibial components, positioning of 157*f*
Femoral and tibial surfaces 62
Femoral artery, descending genicular branch of 7
Femoral bone cuts, anteroposterior 54
Femoral canal 51, 52
  blocking 58
  placement of bony block for 59*f*
  removal of jigs 59*f*
Femoral component 168, 169
  rotation 54
  sagittal alignment 144*f*
  sizing 54
Femoral condyles 167
  posterior 88*f*
Femoral cut, anterior 55*f*
Femoral cuts 56
  posterior 55*f*
Femoral entry with drill 52*f*

Femoral implant 69*f*, 170*f*
periphery of 69*f*
templating of 42*f*
trial 58
Femoral intercondylar notch, excision of 57*f*
Femoral jig placement in flexion 103*f*
Femoral osteophytes 75*f*
Femoral preparation, use of robotic burr for 165*f*
Femoral rotation 168
Femoral sizing jig 54, 54*f*
Femoral surface with bone cement 69*f*
Femur 5
anatomical axis 11
mechanical axis 11
on tibia rectangularizes flexion gap 14*f*
Fixed bearing 130, 130*f*, 130*t*
implants 130
Fixed valgus knees 84
Flexed knee deformity 85*f*
corrected 89*f*
correction of 89*f*
X-rays of 86*f*
Flexion-extension gap in
extension 56*f*
flexion 56*f*
Focal metaphyseal defect 91
Foot pumps 121
Fracture
arthritic joints 28
type of 126
Functional scoring chart 46*f*
Fused knee 28, 100
planned 101*f*
pose excessive challenges 100

G

Gap
assessment and alignment 56
balancing technique 164
Genu recurvatum 95
Genu valgum 95
Geometric knee prosthesis 151
Glass-filled polyamide 169
Good operation theater environment 33*f*
Grafted bone defects 94*f*

H

Hamstring
muscle strength 36
strengthening and stretching 111
Handheld navigation works 158
Heart rate, continuous monitoring of 105
Hip abductor 111
Hip-knee-ankle axis 168
Hohman's retractors, placement of 49

I

Iliopsoas strengthening 111
Iliotibial band, anterior fibers of 80
Implant
component inventory 32
durability 136
evolution of 139, 146, 149, 151
position of 70*f*, 72*f*
systems and designs 17
Implantation and reduction, trial 58
Infection 35, 135
Inferior vena cava filters 119
Inflammatory arthropathies 36
Informed consent 37, 39*f*
Instrumentation set inventory 32
Intensive care unit 37
Intercondylar notch, preservation of 151*f*
Intermittent pneumatic compression device 118
Intra-articular fracture 27
Intramedullary femoral jig 53*f*
Intramedullary jig 52
removed 53*f*
Intramedullary rod 53
Intramedullary rotary planning tool 73
Intramedullary stems, use of 94

J

Joint
- assessment, preoperative 36
- kinematics and balance 158
- line obliquity angle 12
- stability in varus-valgus 56
- with trial femoral implant 59*f*

K

Keel punch 61, 62*f*
Kinematic 11, 16
- alignment techniques 168
- prosthesis 2
- rotating hinge 1
- rotating hinge knee prosthesis 2*f*

Kissing lesion 142*f*
Knee
- anatomical and mechanical axes of 12*f*
- anterior
  - muscular anatomy of 7*f*
  - part of 143
- anteromedial nervous anatomy of 9*f*
- arthritic 138
- arthroplasty
  - classification of combined partial 150*f*
  - combined partial 149
  - first resection 1
- bending 111
  - protocol 111*f*
- classification, coronal plane alignment of 12
- coronal plane alignment of 13*f*
- grab 143
- implant assembly 170*f*
- joint, bones of 170*f*
- menisci and ligaments, cross-sectional anatomy 6*f*
- motion 11
- normal 11
- posterior nervous anatomy of 9*f*
- posteromedial corner of 19
- rotation of 2*f*
- stability and alignment 60
- surgical anatomy of 7*f*
- unstable 28
- with total knee arthroplasty prosthesis 15
- X-ray of 104*f*, 126*f*

Knee replacement
- bilateral 113
- computer-assisted 16*f*
- contraindication for 30*f*
- extended indications for 29*f*

Knee scoring 36, 44
Knee Society Clinical Rating System 44
Knee society pain 46*f*
Knee society radiological scoring chart 47*f*
Knee society score 44
Knee society scoring questionnaire 45*f*

L

Laminar air flow systems 31, 34*f*, 133. 135
- used in operation theaters 135*f*

Lateral distal femoral angle 13
Lateral epicondyle slide osteotomy 26
Lateral femoral condyle defect 81*f*
Lateral popliteal nerve 9
Laxity 48
Ligament balancing methods 10
Ligaments 5
- medial collateral 6, 74, 96, 100
- posterior capsule 6
- posterior cruciate
  - retaining 127, 127*t*
  - sacrificing 127, 127*t*
- anterior cruciate 5, 6, 96, 152
- lateral collateral 6, 25, 96
- posterior cruciate 5, 6, 77, 81, 96, 127, 128

Light emitting diodes 155
Low contact stress design 4*f*
Low-dose unfractionated heparin 118
Lower limb, mechanical axis of 11
Low-molecular-weight heparin 115*f*, 119, 144

M

Menisci 49
 and fat pad, excision of 50*f*
Metal-backed tibial component 139*f*
Microfractures 138
Midvastus 21
 approach 21
Minimally invasive
 approaches 26
 incision vis-à-vis standard incision 26*f*
Mobile bearing 130, 130*t*
 tibial inserts 130, 130*f*
Muscle forces 6

N

Neural damage 88
Neuromuscular disorders 95
Neurovascular
 anatomy 6
 complications 122
 implications 10
Neutral alignment, restoration of 94
Nonsteroidal anti-inflammatory drugs 36, 138
Notch 56

O

One-finger test 143
Operation theater 31, 37, 40*f*
Osteoarthritis 138, 152
Osteoarticular allograft 138
Osteochondral autograft 138
Osteology 5
Osteolysis 124
Osteoperiosteal sleeve 25*f*
Osteophytes 75
 excised 61
 removal of 129
 removal of 88*f*
Osteotome
 and hammer, removal of posterior osteophytes 58*f*
 posteromedial release with 76*f*
Osteotomy joint line, double level 102*f*
Oxford knee score 44

P

Pain
 and inflammation 88
 control 106
 management 106
 scoring 36
 site of 143
Painted and draped extremity 40*f*
Parapatellar approach 79
Parapatellar approach, medial 19
Patella 5, 61, 128, 170*f*
 position 5
 preparation 61
 replacement 129
 thickness 62
Patellaplasty 64, 66*f*, 129*f*
Patellar button 17, 64*f*
 implantation, level for 64*f*
 trial 64
Patellar
 clamp 67*f*
 eversion 51
 implant undersurface 67*f*
 jaw clamp 62
  holding patella 63*f*
 jig 63
 nonresurfacing 128, 128*t*
 osteophytes, excision of 63*f*
 prosthesis 129*f*
 resurfacing 128, 128*t*
 subluxation 51
 surface 66*f*
 thickness using vernier calipers 63*f*
 tracking 72*f*, 87, 97
Patellofemoral
 alignment 13
 arthroplasty 148*f*
 crepitus 148
 implant design 147*f*
 instability 125
Patellofemoral joint arthroplasty 145, 146
 evolution of implants 146
 indications and contraindications 147
 prosthesis 147*f*
Patellofemoral joint, extensive degeneration of 146*f*

Patellofemoral osteoarthritis 145, 147*f*
Patellofemoral tracking 22, 61, 65*f*, 77, 83
Peripatellar synovium, light cauterization of 63*f*
Peripheral defects 91
Periprosthetic fracture 126
Photopolymers 169
Polyarticular disease 36
Poly carbonate 169
Poly tibial component 4*f*
Polycentric knee 151
Polyethylene tibial component 139*f*
Polylactic acid 169
Popliteus tendon 6
Posterolateral capsule, piecrust lengthening of 81*f*
Postorgan transplant 137
Postpulsatile lavage 67*f*
Precrust lengthening, lateral approach 23*f*
Print metallic shape 169*f*
Prophylaxis
  primary 120
  secondary 120
Prosthesis, condylar type of 86
Prosthetic
  instability 96
  materials 4
Protruding medial tibial, excision of 75*f*
Proximal tibial
  and distal femoral cuts 159*f*
  angle, medial 13
  bone cut 51
  cut 52*f*, 80*f*
    3D printed specific jigs for 167*f*
  osteotomy 138
Pulmonary embolism 35, 114, 121
Pulsatile lavage 67*f*
Pulsatile lavage system 33*f*, 133*f*, 133, 137

Q

Q-angle 14*f*
Quadriceps 36
  setting exercises 110*f*
  strengthening 110
  turndown
    Insall's modification of 24
    procedure 23
  V-Y plasty 23*f*
  weakness 95

R

Radiological
  assessment 41
  evaluation 41*f*
Radiology and templating 41
Ranawat's jig 54
  used for sizing 55*f*
Range of motion 59, 134, 152
  assessment of balance in 164*f*
  knee 158
Reciprocating saw, cutting of notch with 57*f*
Recovery room
  position in 105
  postoperative 105*f*
Rectus snip 24
  procedure 24*f*
Recurvatum, cause of 95
Recurvatum deformity 95
  correction of 99*f*
Recurvatum knee deformities, corrected 99*f*
Recurvatum right knee deformity 95*f*, 96*f*
  under anesthesia 96*f*
Red flags 109
Registration process 157*f*
Repicci unicompartmental knee prosthesis 139*f*
Respiratory distress 109
Retinacular closure, medial 73*f*
Retinaculum 71
Rheumatoid arthritis 95, 137
Robert-Jones compression bandage 73*f*
Robot-assisted bone resections 164
Robotic assistance, functional alignment 168*f*
Robotic-assisted 43
  surgery 95, 160
Robotic engineer 163

S

Sclerotic bone surfaces 61
Semimembranosus, 6
Semitendinosus 6
Side support with tourniquet 49*f*
Skin incision 49, 71
Smith–Peterson took molds 167
Smooth patellar surface postpatellaplasty 66*f*
Soft tissue 5
- balancing 76, 80, 86, 97, 103
- envelope 168
- hypermobility 99
- knowledge of 5
- release 50

Spherocentric knee 1
Spinal anesthesia 144
Stair climbing 111
Standard skin midline incision 19
Staple removal 112*f*, 144
Stemmed tibial implants 94*f*
Stick aided walking 111
Stretching 110
Subluxation, increased risk of 123
Subvastus 19
Suction apparatus 31, 33*f*
Superficial and deep dissection 50*f*
Superficial dissection, standard approach 20*f*
Supracondylar periprosthetic femoral fracture 126*f*
Supracondylar region 126
Surgical technique
- bone defect management 90
- flexion deformity 85
- fused knee takedown 100
- recurvatum deformity 95
- standard knee 49
- valgus deformity 78
- varus deformity 74

Surgical workflow 156, 162
Suture removal 113

T

Tegaderm dressing and drain 73*f*
Three-D printed prototypes 170*f*
Thrombi quite, presence of 114
Thromboprophylaxis 119, 137
- initiation of 119
- role of 137
- update 114

Thrombus generation, cascade of 114*f*
Tibia 5
- anatomical axis 11
- drill hole in 62*f*

Tibial
- anatomical axis 5
- and femoral array positioning 164
- component 65, 168
  - backside wear on 124*f*
  - slope 144*f*
- corner, posteromedial, complete exposure of 50*f*
- cut with stylus, level of 51*f*
- implant 42*f*
  - impaction of 68*f*
  - periphery of 68*f*
- insert liner 170*f*
- jig placement 102*f*
- nerve 8
- plateau
  - contained defect in 92*f*
  - defect in 92*f*
  - managed with metal wedge 93*f*
- preparation 61
  - jig, placement of 62*f*
- sizing 51
  - with trial tibial tray 52*f*
- slope, posterior 12*f*
- surface 50*f*
- tray 170*f*
  - final insert placed 71*f*
  - rotational alignment of 61*f*
  - trial 58
  - with insertion device 71*f*

Tibial tubercle 5, 102*f*
- osteotomy 24, 25*f*
  - fixation 104*f*

Titanium 169
Titanium-aluminum-vanadium alloy 169
Toilet training 111
Total condylar prosthesis 1, 3*f*
Total knee arthroplasty 27*f*, 47, 116, 134, 138, 151, 152, 162, 163

anatomically aligned 15
bicruciate retaining 150, 151, 152, 152*t*
computer software for 163*f*
computer-assisted surgery, 154
economics of 133
implants 17*f*
instrumentation sets 18*f*
kinematically aligned 15
mechanically aligned 15
personalized 166
prosthesis
axes reconstruction with 15*f*, 16*f*
dislocated 124*f*
robotic-assisted 166
robots in 161
roentgenographic evaluation and scoring system 47
ROSA system for 162*f*
surgery 17, 27, 35, 121, 136*f*
late complication 123*f*
typical X-rays of 28*f*
Total knee components, cementless fixation of 72
Total knee replacement 43
revision 125*f*
Tourniquet 71, 137
and drains, use of 131
Transportation to recovery room 105
Trial tibial tray, alignment rod placed 60*f*
Tricompartmental disease 142
Trochlear dysplasia 147*f*

U

Ultra-clean filters 135
Uncemented 130, 130*t*
Unicompartment knee arthroplasty 28, 131*f*, 138, 140, 166
implants, types of 139
medial 21
radiographic evaluation of 144*f*
surgery, newer tools in 145*f*
Unicompartmental interpositional implant 138
Unicondylar knee replacement 138

V

Vacuum mixers 136
Vacuum mixing device, basic 137*f*
Valgus angle 53*f*
Valgus correction 9
Valgus deformity 78, 79*f*
corrected 83*f*, 84*f*
under anesthesia, severity and correctability of 80*f*
Valgus knee 82
Valgus knee deformities 78*f*
X-rays of 79*f*
Valgus stress, stability with trial implants 60*f*
Varicose ulcers 35
Varus deformity 74
preoperative 77*f*
severe 76*f*
Varus knee deformity 74*f*
X-rays of 75*f*
Varus knees, severe 91*f*
Varus stress, stability with trial implants 60*f*
Varus-valgus
balance 59
stability 57*f*
Vascular anatomy 8*f*
Venous thromboembolism, perioperative prophylaxis of 116
Visual analogue scale 113
Vitamin K
antagonist 118
anticoagulants 122
V-Y quadricepsplasty 24, 104*f*

W

Walker aided ambulation 113
Walking with walker 108*f*
aided support 111
Wound
closure 71, 77
lavage 64

Z

Zimmer 141*f*